Praise

D

Assistant Professor, School of Nursing, McGill
University

"This book will convince everyone that
caring, skilled nurses remain the cornerstone of
our health care system."

Victor W. Cummings
Actor/Broadcaster

"A pleasant read but hard to tear oneself
away. Author Lillian R. Tymchuk's compilation
of stories, anecdotes, thoughts, and revelations
tugs at the whole range of human emotions. I
laughed, loved, cried, mused and meditated. I'm
sure all these very professional nurses who told
their stories did so with a progressive sense of
hesitation, conviction, pride and relict."

"Congratulations to this brilliant author
for allowing the reading public to be privy to
many suppressed experiences they would
otherwise never know."

Pray for Nurse, Hear You Hear Me

Dr. Bonnie Lee Smith N.Ph.D.

Published by:

Wordstorm Productions Inc.,
Box 49132, 7740 - 18 St SE,
Calgary, Alberta, Canada
T2C 3W5

US address:

Wordstorm Productions Inc.,
1520 3 rd St NW, C-104,
Great Falls, Montana, USA 59404

ISBN: 0-9697756-8-7
Printed in Canada
First printing, May, 1997
Wordstorm Productions Inc.®

Cover art   © Wordstorm Productions Inc. 1997

Cover design: Wordstorm Productions Inc.
                   Perry P. Rose

Wordstorm Editor: Laurie Anne Witwer

Cataloguing in Publication Data

Tymchuk, Lillian, 1943 -
        Nurse: hear you, hear me

ISBN 0-9697756-8-7

        1. Nursing — anecdotes. I. Title.

RT34.T94 1997   610.73   C97-900280-X

Please visit our Web Site at:

http://www.cadvision.com?wordstorm/word1.html

ACKNOWLEDGEMENTS

To the registered nurses in each of the provinces and territories who so generously shared their true nursing experiences, I would like to express my sincere gratitude and appreciation. Others who have been an invigorating and positive influence are the Class of '64 at Hamilton Civic Hospitals, and the many superb nurses and doctors with whom I have had the pleasure of working.

I am especially indebted to my publisher, Perry P. Rose, for his belief in my work along with his considerate, often humorous, support and encouragement throughout this exciting process. Thankyou to editor Laurie Anne Witwer for her meticulous attention to detail, my niece Paula J. Tymchuk for her photographic expertise, to my writing "friends" Robert Neilsen and Myra Woods (thanks for the scintiallating lunches), and to Deborah H. Cassidy, M.S.W., for her invaluable input.

I am very grateful for the love and encouragement from my brothers and their families — Paul and Anna, Walter and Patricia, Paula and Jeff, Michele, Gail, and little Tatyana with her sunshine smile. Special and grateful thanks to my beloved cat "Banjo" for being the perfect writer's cat.

The source of quotations is the Oxford Dictionary of Quotations - Third Editon.

Nursing statistics (1994) are courtesy of the Ontario Nurses' Association.

Nurse

Hear You
Hear Me

Lillian R. Tymchuk, R.N

For my father and mother

Steve and Florence Tymchuk

with love
especially for the Dunnville Days

<u>INTRODUCTION</u>

In this non-fiction book many of the experiences of the registered nurses can best be described as being a powerful moment or epiphany. Poets have described such happenings as "spots of time" or "the best and happiest moments . . . arising unforseen and departing unbidden." These magical moments are magnified and forever remain in the mind as a cherished memory — moments of grace embraced by elegance, moments of sorrow embraced by the need for deeper understanding, moments of amazement embraced by the unknown, and moments of joy and laughter embraced by a sense of gratitued and appreciation.

As a third year nursing student at Hamilton General Hosital in the early '60's, I worked nights on a medical floor and enjoyed many breakfasts with a head nurse who worked permanent nights in Emergency. The exciting stories about her shifts in Emerg fascinated me and I knew that was where I wanted to work. I was hooked.

The powerful stories continued and nurses in all areas of health care said, "Someone should write these down!" That is how and why this book came to be.

The issue of confidentiality had to be dealt with while maintaining the integrity of the stories. This was of tremendous concern to all the nurses whom I interviewed. As a result, nurses and patients have not been identified.

While health care across the whole of the nation is undergoing drastic changes, this book is in no way a definitive comment on current political or economic transformations. It neither endorses nor denies any specific treatments. Rather, it is a celebration of the professional registered nurse and the care she provides at the bedside of her patient.

ONE

THE NITTY GRITTY OF
PATIENT ADVOCACY
- ℞ - ℞ - ℞ -

Catullus gives you warmest thanks,
And he the worst of poets ranks;
As much the worst of bards confessed,
As you of advocates the best.
Catullus, 87-54? BC

The nitty-gritty life and work of the professional registered nurse takes place at the bedside, where the heart and soul of the profession always have been and always will be.

To be an advocate is to plead for another, to speak in favour of, defend, recommend, support. During the Crimean War, a war in which more men died of disease than of wounds suffered on the battlefield, Florence Nightingale greatly reduced death amongst the soldiers by introducing strict sanitary measures and nursing standards. Florence Nightingale, patient advocate.

That patients require advocates is sad. That patients have nurses as advocates is splendid. In each of the following accounts, the theme that is lovingly embroidered into the tapestry of modern multi-disciplinary care is that of the nurse as patient advocate.

WEEBLES-WOBBLES
- R - R - R -

Cindy is one of 30,746 nurses in British Columbia. She specializes in dialysis for kids and treasures each day she spends with them as they fight for their lives. Here is Cindy's story.

We dialyze kids from age three weeks to nineteen years — the older ones go to an adult centre. One day I had an experience scary enough to make my heart jump into my mouth.

Our kids are generally quite small, and two-year-old Howie was no exception, weighing in at eleven kilos. These kids are small for their age, because their growth and development are much slower and their bones don't elongate normally.

Howie fought every day from the moment he was born with no complaint. He arrived with only one dysplastic kidney and that had to be removed, so he needed dialysis. He spent the first year and a half of his life in the hospital, during which he was on peritoneal dialysis — that didn't work too well. Then he was put on renal dialysis till he was three. We watched him blossom as he came in four times every week. He wanted to walk and talk, and to say all of our names. He was "our boy."

He was so funny but he knew exactly what he was doing. He would entertain us for hours, laughing, singing, and dancing with his arms, the way his mother taught him. Howie was a very small but extremely active two-year-old.

He had a yellow box full of eight Weebles-Wobbles, funny little egg-shaped men. Push them down and they pop back up. He named each of them after one of us, and he wouldn't allow us to mix them up. I would say one was Katie or Laura, and he would correct me, "No, that's Luba." He charmed us all.

Howie was starting to eat shortly after his second birthday. When these kids don't eat, we use stomach tubes to feed them. Dialysis patients get this metallic taste in their mouth and are somewhat anorexic. That's why it's important for kids between two and four to get their calories. You're between a rock and a hard place, because they need the calories but they can't have the fluid. They can't have potassium. They can't have sodium. They can't have calcium. It's a dietitian's nightmare. This was a real battle for us and Howie's family.

There are a lot of lines — or tubing — associated with dialysis. We have certain lines we use for

5

older kids, and others we use for the younger ones. The ironic thing is the adult ones come with a fail-safe lock, but not the ones for the kids.

Consequently, we always had to carefully cross-tape the two pieces of tubing together for the little kids, since it often took three hours for dialysis.

One morning Howie was sitting up in his crib being dialyzed, laughing and playing games, with a little blue and white blanket around his skinny shoulders. All of a sudden he fell back and slouched into the corner, a sickly hue permeating his body.

I pulled the blanket back. The two lines had become disconnected, and blood was pouring all over the crib. The two separate ends of tubing, that I had so carefully taped together, flopped around wildly as if they had lives of their own.

Howie was losing blood so rapidly there wasn't time to put new lines in. Within seconds, he arrested. We called a code.

"GIVE ME THE LINE NOW!"

We put the lines back together as quickly as we could, in one second, in two seconds ... it seemed like an eternity.

Normal sterile procedure had to be bypassed, but at length our nephrologist put the pump back on and gave Howie the blood volume he so desperately needed. After it was all over we were reminded how fast these kids can code with any blood loss.

Howie's mother, who rarely left his side, had taken a break when all this happened and we were thankful, because we were close to her. She would have understood that it was an accident, but the experience wouldn't have done her any good.

For a while Howie was fine. But he could not live ad infinitum on dialysis, and he was put on the waiting list for a kidney transplant.

Two weeks before Christmas he got his transplant, but there were problems. His blood pressure was sky high, which in itself was not unusual. But he had an episode that was a questionable bleed, and possibly either a seizure or aspiration of fluid into his lungs. After that there was nothing left. Howie was brain dead. He died within a short time.

His mother had to deal with the guilt of having accepted the transplant, for saying yes to the phone call offering a cadaver kidney, even though it was Howie's only chance for survival.

All the nurses from our outpatient dialysis unit and twenty-something nurses from the nephrology ward attended his funeral. Howie was a special little boy.

THE DEATH BOOK
- R - R - R -

In the process of providing and receiving nursing care, nurse and patient often subtly change, in the same way the colours of the rainbow blur and blend into each other.

Sometimes the line between living and dying gets blurred also, and dedicated nurses such as Norman in

Ontario try to ease the transition — successfully at times and less so at other times, but always with care and compassion.

The place I work is considered a free-standing hospice and is exclusively for people in the end stages of AIDS. The nursing perspective includes what we're doing here, how we've changed, and some of the struggles we've had. We're trying to deliver the same quality of care despite financial restrictions and a change in philosophy at an upper level.

When we first opened our philosophy of good care included two main points — a person never died in pain, and a person never died alone. Over the years we've come to realize that's not always possible. One of the most disturbing things for nurses is having someone die in a great deal of pain.

At the nurses' station we have what is called the Death Book, in which we list everyone who has died here, and something about their dying. There are three books, but only the first and half of the second have entries. After that it peters out. There are no more entries. There are only names and dates and blank pages. The deaths that stand out are the ones where a lot of pain was involved. We may have become inured to death. It's like being in a war where the ordinary death doesn't stand out, just the extraordinary one.

Sometimes we sit around in the nursing station collectively as front-line staff nurses and question — what are we really doing here now? Have we become hardened? Have we become indifferent? Doesn't this touch us anymore? I think we particularly notice this when we reflect back on when we first started several years ago.

Many of us have close ties to the gay community. Although we come from different walks of life, all of the nurses here have experienced loss in their lives, know what it's like to be marginalized in some way, what it's like to stand up for one's rights, and how to be a community advocate. That's a commonality we share.

Certainly with the number of deaths we've had the actual nature of the disease is changing somewhat. When people first came here, their first or second bout of pneumonia would kill them. We had time to be at the bedside to do all those comforting things, to have the sheets turned down just so, to sit and talk with the family, and to listen.

Now, people with AIDS are living longer. They're surviving their fourth and fifth bouts because of medication. But MAI, one of the diseases associated with AIDS, has a devastating effect on the gastrointestinal and nervous systems, and can lead to blindness and dementia.

We're dealing with people who are agitated, anxious, stressed out, and difficult to deal with. The solution to such a problem in the usual setting is chemical or physical restraint, but that goes against our philosophy because it's undignifying. We feel we can support them through this, and we know our approach works.

Trying to deliver the same quality of care now is much more difficult and frustrating. We feel we're giving hospital quality of care — meaning that our staffing is at hospital level. We do the tasks, but we can't be there like we should. It's getting tougher to deliver on our motto, "Giving Compassion a Home." We may need to develop a work- smart program.

On a personal level, I occasionally find myself speeding up and becoming task oriented — there's laser treatment to do, a couple of baths, and someone down the hall is a total feed. Before I know it, I'm so revved up and focused on tasks that I fly into the room and busily do these things, while my mind is on tasks still awaiting.

I had the privilege of attending a hospice seminar in Britain where I heard a saying that made a big impression on me, "Hurry Hurts, Calmness Heals." I try to make this part of my daily routine but it is troublesome.

For instance, there was Danny, who had about a month left to live. He was in a double room, wholly dependent. His dementia and fevers had him calling out loudly, getting up, stumbling about the room, and disturbing his roommate.

Two successive roommates couldn't handle him either. They complained and were upset, wondering how we could control his behaviour. It was worrisome.

We moved Danny closer to the nursing station so we could be there to intervene promptly if he fell or tried to get out of bed.

His latest roommate, Gerald, was on what we call respite care. He seemed to be well, was good-looking and personable, and easygoing with his care. "Whenever you can get to me is okay," he would say.

One night, Danny had been agitating the whole shift, while Gerald remained calm. As I made my rounds there was no sound coming from the room. I thought Danny probably had fallen out of bed and I'd find him unconscious on the floor. When I went in, there was Danny sitting on the side of his bed. Gerald sat beside him, supporting him by the shoulders, feeding him an orange popsicle.

Seeing this was so profound for us because at the time we were undergoing yet another structural change. Nursing was really stressed out and we were not in a happy head space about the care we were giving or the work load we had. Yet, here was compassion right in front of our noses. Gerald had every right to complain about his noisy roommate, but he chose not to. He saw an alternative way, and that taught me a lesson.

We have difficulty sometimes with how we're presented to the public. We're not angels of compassion, we're people trying to do our job. It is a struggle at times, particularly when there's been a lot of death, or a difficult death without a good resolution — when we don't have time to talk over how we feel about it, or we're blithely told, "You did the best you could under the circumstances," and it's left at that.

It's important to process these feelings and to talk about where the sense of failure came from. Did we

11

feel we were supported? What can we do when we encounter this situation the next time?

A predicament I can think of quite clearly concerns a fellow named Richard, who was dying, and his parents were in denial of his sexuality and of his dying. His mother would come in and intimate that the other residents sitting around the lounge had done something to deserve this illness, but not her son. People stopped coming into the lounge when she was there.

As Richard became increasingly ill, she became more frantic. She felt we weren't feeding him properly, so she would bring him meals from home. The fact was that he was nauseated and vomiting all the time. She would push the food down and it would readily come up. We would go in there and clean him up and she'd pick up a spoon and start on him all over again.

Despite repeated suggestions like, "This is not working, please give him a rest," she was driven to feed him because part of her culture dictated that if you can get food into someone, then they've got a chance of pulling through. All the education we provided to her on what AIDS was doing to his gut just wasn't helping.

Pain was another big issue. In her eyes we were aiding and abetting his death with morphine. He would be lying on his bed in severe pain and I would come in with the break-through morphine. She would knock it out of my hand or physically hold me back, despite my explanations.

12

The counsellors couldn't help either. The mother would lock herself in the bathroom and scream. The circumstances were stressful and complex.

There was an intense family meeting just before Richard died. Again we explained how we were trying to control his pain. Surprisingly, this time the mother said she could trust us and felt that we were working for her son.

But when the crisis came and he was dying, she utterly dissembled, and became overwrought. The screaming started again, and she yanked us away from the bed when we tried to medicate him. At one point she screamed at me, "Go ahead and give it to him. He's dead now anyway!"

But Richard was alive and he could hear. I can't begin to describe the sense of futility I felt. There was no sense of peace in the room. It was not a good dying.

We were relieved when at last he did die, both for him and for ourselves, because we wouldn't have his mother to contend with anymore. I didn't think I could ever work with that cultural background again, but now I know I would at least try.

Another resident, named Ludvig, was from the States. His dying was arduous because he was raised as a Catholic and he'd been brought up to believe he was sinful because of his sexual orientation. Peace continued to elude him, even after the sacrament of healing from his priest.

Near the end he lapsed into his mother tongue and couldn't comprehend anything we said to him in English. We wondered why he lingered on.

He was in such psychic pain. At first we thought it was physical pain, but all the Dilaudid and Morphine we gave him didn't touch him. His brow creased and he moaned incessantly, obviously troubled.

One evening his friends told me that Ludvig had worked as a nurses' aide in a geriatrics' home, and his care was compassionate, gentle, and thorough. The patients looked forward to seeing him because of the sense of dignity he brought to their lives.

I contacted an interpreter who translated into German for me what Ludvig had done with his life — his kindness, his humaneness, and the fact that God would welcome him when he died because of his loving care and compassion for these elderly people. We read this to him repeatedly over the next two hours, in our fractured German.

Ludvig's brow relaxed, and his moaning ceased. His spiritual fear seemed to ease, and shortly thereafter, he died peacefully.

Therapeutic touch can help in the same way. Another resident who was dying was radically bitter because this was going to be his last Christmas.

When I came in to do therapeutic touch, he was wound up as tightly as a coiled spring. Afterward, he said "thank you" in a strained, controlled voice.

Ten minutes later he exploded. He lashed out at his partner, "It's going to be a right merry Christmas for you with me being gone," and he burst into tears. His lover held him and rocked him. Somehow we enabled that emotion to happen.

I have a sense that we're evolving, and as nurses we're going to have to be better educated. How we deal with the challenge of continuing in a hospice mode remains to be seen.

A DIFFERENT FOCUS
- ℞ - ℞ - ℞ -

Deborah specializes in mental health in Prince Edward Island. "I used to love working in acute care," she says, "but all the emphasis there was on the illness. The focus in mental health is entirely different."

I work in community mental health, with people just like you and me, although recently I looked after the long- term, mentally ill clients.

The majority of clients I provide care for never see a psychiatrist and are not admitted to hospital — they're working people. Primarily I see single mothers and women with relationship problems. Most are referred by family doctors and it's getting difficult to keep up with the steadily increasing numbers.

Instead of being labelled as crazy, by virtue of seeing a psychiatrist, our clients feel we help when we say, "What and how you're feeling is normal, given all your stressors. We're not here to make light of what you are, or to say you're sick, but rather to help you discover what you can do to remove some of the stressors."

This approach is much more satisfying and becomes a learning and growing experience for both of us. I can say to my clients, "You give me much more than I ever give you."

One recent crisis had to do with sexual abuse. Marilyn, a young mother, became hysterical when she realized her common-law husband was abusing Lisa, her six-year-old daughter.

Marilyn was a "walk-in" who initially didn't present her problem openly. She kept insisting she was depressed, but after half an hour she began to open up.

She first suspected major problems with sexual abuse when Lisa began exhibiting a disturbing change in her behaviour. Once a happy, carefree little girl who loved to play with her friends, Lisa gradually became withdrawn, fearful and sad. She would cry whenever her mother went out even if it was only for a short time.

Lisa began to visibly cringe whenever the common-law husband was around and eventually refused to stay in the same room with him. Nonetheless she was unable to verbalize the traumatic events taking place in her home, even to her own mother.

Eventually Marilyn figured out what was going on but she didn't know how to deal with the situation. She had difficulty in believing that something so horrendous could be happening to her little girl at the hand of someone she thought she loved. She ended up kicking the man out and charging him. I had no choice but to get Social Services involved.

I saw her a couple of times in the first week and several times after that. Fortunately, she had a wealth of family support and understanding, so she was well off in that respect. One of my colleagues looked after her daughter, because I don't work with kids under sixteen. Both Marilyn and Lisa worked hard on coming to terms with a difficult situation and now they are doing reasonably well.

In our clinic there are social workers and psychologists. We do the initial assessment, and if we think a psychiatrist is required, we call him in.

We've been trying to work with school children. People have to build more on their self-esteem when they are six years old and in grade one, rather than when they are forty-two, have had three losses, and wonder why they're falling apart. There is a drastic need both to promote mental health and to prevent mental illnesses and we are striving toward attainment of these goals in our clinic.

HEAR YOU, HEAR ME
- ℞ - ℞ - ℞ -

Marion, a nurse from Saskatchewan, says she doesn't like the direction nursing is taking. "I'm glad I'm on the going-out end of nursing rather than the coming-in end, because I don't think I could handle the new philosophy."

The nuns who trained me said the only reason we were here was to take care of patients, to give patient care, to give grieving patients moral, emotional, and religious support, and they meant every word of it.

They taught us that hearing was the first sense to come back and the last one to leave, and to be careful what we said. This has played on my mind many times.

Any operating rooms I've worked in are all the same. The doctors get the patient to sleep and then the jokes start. It's happy time.

In one OR we had a patient who was a single, professional lady in her mid-forties and considered to be very prim and proper. She was having a minor gynecological operation. As soon as the anaesthetist put her to sleep, her doctor began to make obnoxious and salacious remarks about her. Always at his outrageous and reprehensible best when his patients were asleep and unable to fend for themselves, this doctor laughed and chortled uncontrollably throughout the short procedure, delighting in his sarcastic witticisms, all of which were at the expense of his trusting patient. As usual, he ignored our protests.

When she woke up, I was relieving in the recovery room. The first thing she said to me was, "He's been my doctor for many years, but not anymore. I'm going to see my lawyer the minute I get out of here. I heard every disgusting word he said."

When stroke patients first come around, they say people scream at them and think that just because they can't talk, they can't hear, and they must be stupid.

People talk down to them like they're two years old. We, as nurses can't let that happen.

READY FOR TAKE-OFF
- R - R - R -

Brenda is one of 5,554 nurses in Newfoundland/Labrador. Her nursing experiences are unique to her own little island, which is an hour from the mainland by ferry.

We have had some harrowing times trying to transfer critically ill patients to the mainland, especially in the winter.

Our small cottage hospital services the whole island, which encompasses ten or eleven communities. This is a great area for a new grad to get experience. We're open round the clock in emergency, but last Christmas we were down to one doctor on call and he was here for three weeks by himself. We have no specialists here on a regular basis.

One foggy morning following report, a fifteen-year-old girl came in, in active labour, tying up the other RN. Within minutes we got an urgent call concerning a woman who sounded sick, so we dispatched the ambulance, which is situated next to the hospital.

The RNA took care of the floor while I rushed down to emergency with the two doctors. When the woman arrived, the doctors suspected an abdominal aortic aneurysm. We did the primary care and transfused her with blood. In the middle of all this, the young girl upstairs was delivering, so one of the doctors ran to deliver the baby.

I arranged to transfer our patient to the mainland and soon the helicopter landed on the hospital's landing pad. She was conscious throughout and was fairly stable when the resident and I loaded her into the helicopter. Despite dense fog we took off for the airstrip, a twenty minute flight.

She remained relatively stable while we made our noisy landing. We loaded her into a waiting airplane for the flight to the mainland, and readied for takeoff. We never did lift off. Half way down the runway she died.

We returned by ambulance through the fog and took her down to the hospital morgue. Her body was later transferred off the island for an autopsy.

Back in the hospital, I had to catch up on my charting. The other nurse, who had stayed overtime, went home, leaving myself and one RNA on duty.

I received a call from a woman who said her teenage daughter had a severe headache and she was bringing her in. Within moments this hysterical lady ran in. Her daughter was in the back seat of the car, semi-conscious, foaming at the mouth, pupils dilated. The doctor, who was walking down the path toward the hospital, ran over when he saw what was happening.

He's a big, tall man. I'm only about a hundred pounds, but we managed to get her into the ER. After examining her he diagnosed a subarachnoid hemorrhage.

We started IVs and gave her medications. She had to be transferred out immediately, but by this time the fog had rolled in again and was so dense that the helicopter could not get through.

We contacted air search and rescue, who arrived smartly. The girl did not survive, despite the transfer. She was brain dead. What a day!

Non-emergency patients go by ferry when it's appropriate, e.g., for elective surgery or further tests like ultrasound.

It's not unusual for us to get weathered out. We've been isolated on the island for up to a week with no mail service and no food coming in. The ferry we have now is small and has to have an ice-breaker with her at all times. We're hoping to get one that can hold more cars and has ice-breaking capacity.

Our island may be small but we work hard at providing the best care possible for our patients, who really are our friends and families. Besides making sure we have the required technical skills and caring, healing hands, we also have to secure the most effective mode of transportation for our patients.

A COUPLE OF SCREWS
- R - R - R -

Some emergency nurses find humour in practically every situation and always have a joke to lighten the mood. Bobby Jo, to whom other nurses flock for the joke of the day, is one such delightful Ontario nurse.

Was this really me inspecting a Cheyenne and a Navaho? It was all part of a course meant to prepare me for air ambulance transfers. I practised putting out different types of fires — oil, gas, and plain wood.

Two pilots usually accompany us and the planes hold no more than five people as passengers. The Cheyenne has room for only one stretcher while the Navaho can hold two.

I completed the required orientation and got my first call several weeks later. Now I am considered medical cabin crew, which means I am responsible for the patient and for the people who accompany the patient. I'm a glorified stewardess in many ways but I do have the final say regarding takeoff if there is a question as to whether a patient is stable enough to fly.

I was asked to transfer a neo-natal infant to northern Ontario. Because it was my first flight, I was nervous and didn't want to make any mistakes. I arrived at the airport the required half hour prior to leaving, with a few minutes to spare.

My internal inspection of the plane assured me all needed supplies were there and I waited impatiently on the tarmac. Soon the ambulance roared up, and out came a nurse with a tiny infant who had major problems — cerebral palsy and a predisposition to seizures.

We hooked up the incubator and secured it to the stretcher, and I did my little spiel about seatbelts, emergency exits, and no smoking. I had never worn headgear before and it was fascinating to listen to all the gibber between the pilots and the tower.

We took off. My anxiety level was at an all-time high as I checked and re-checked the baby, and made sure my equipment was intact and operational. The day was beautiful, spectacular really.

I had never been to northern Ontario before and was amazed to see how, from high up, the land looked similar to pictures I had seen of the Northwest Territories with its numerous bodies of water and trees. The flight was smooth and uneventful and my anxieties gradually faded. The baby showed no signs of seizures and rewarded me with a sweet smile. Her nurse relinquished her to a waiting nurse once we arrived at our destination.

With a sigh of relief I prepared for the return flight. Once we were airborne, I heard the pilot and the co-pilot saying something about losing pressure, but I didn't know what they meant.

I thought I heard a small hissing sound and the other nurse heard something as well. In the meantime, the co-pilot came back and explained that we were losing cabin pressure, and asked us to help find a leak, probably the root of the problem.

We unbuckled our seatbelts and crawled around on the floor, searching for the leak with our fingers. I ran my hand on the track where the chairs normally sat, and the noise stopped. One of the screws in the track had become unpried, and this was where our air leak was. No need for concern — we just lost a couple of screws.

DEGREE, PRIORITY, AND PLACE
- ℞ - ℞ - ℞ -

Annette, an OR nurse in Quebec, was faced with minimal staff and a lineup of gravely ill patients requiring immediate surgery.

Last winter we had a major snowstorm, serious enough to make driving dangerous, especially across the bridge. Although my home is near the hospital, I didn't want to chance the hazardous drive, and the bus couldn't secure enough traction to make it up the hill.

I slid down one street and trudged up the next. Traffic was bumper-to-bumper and it took me an hour of tramping through the snow to get to work.

When I arrived in the OR at four-fifteen, we couldn't start any cases — five nurses had called in sick because of the snowstorm, leaving myself and two others.

On the OR list we had three cases requiring emergency surgery. The first was a forty-year-old man requiring a coronary bypass and was an emergency transfer from another hospital. The second was an elderly lady in the ER who had slipped in the snow, fracturing her left hip. The third was a young woman with a complete bowel obstruction in our ICU.

The surgeons wanted to open two operating rooms, but this was impossible with only three nurses. There wouldn't be anybody in charge, and there wasn't anyone I could call in.

Everything was done in priority. The anesthetist and myself, as the nurse-in-charge, made the decisions in a joint effort. The surgeons had no say, because without the nursing personnel, they could do nothing.

We did the heart first. Everyone was psyched up because of the special circumstances and gave peak performance plus. The operation went like a charm and it actually turned out to be an omen for the rest of the shift. We wheeled our first patient into the recovery room and proceeded with pinning the fractured hip. Smooth. Perfect. Over to the recovery room. Next. Repaired the bowel obstruction. Precise. Faultless.

Rather than feeling exhausted we each felt as if we had been asked to give our best and we had gladly given more. What had started out as individuals practising separate songs became a symphony played in perfect and joyous harmony for the benefit of our patients. This was nursing on a higher level, a different plane — the best!

Lillian R. Tymchuk, RN

SEVENTY-TWO HOURS
- R - R - R -

Nurse Katharine says, "Nova Scotia winters can be fairly temperate because we're by the water, but there's an exception to every rule."

One night, although the weatherman was predicting a slight storm, the sky was beautiful and clear when I drove in to work. I started what I thought was a normal twelve-hour shift on my ten-bed pediatrics unit. Was I wrong.

In a matter of hours a major blizzard roared through, leaving drifting snow piled in its wake. Soon even the snow ploughs couldn't budge. Everything came to a dead halt.

Only the rare snowmobile was able to navigate, but there aren't many of those around here. No one could get in or out. We were stranded.

In the morning, our skeleton night staff was obliged to stay on. Only three people had made it in, and two were in the housekeeping department.

I was lucky. I was working alone on pediatrics because there were only seven patients and they weren't that bad: three kids with fractures, a tonsillectomy, a croup, an asthmatic, and Dolly, a two-year-old who was seizuring.

Dolly was admitted the evening of the storm, and she was my main concern. We planned to transfer

26

her out for further investigation. Hers was not the usual febrile seizure, and we couldn't determine the cause.

For the first twenty-four hours my adrenaline was pumping like crazy. Everybody was excited because it was like an adventure. We did everything — cooking, serving — it was sheer madness. I believe the correct term is holistic care.

Needless to say, we were barely able to give more than basic care. We gave the medications and did essential baths. It was impossible for nurses to give each other proper breaks, given the limited number of staff.

The snow continued to fall all day, and we stayed on for another twelve-hour night shift. On about the thirtieth hour on duty I could hardly put one foot in front of the other with any degree of steadiness. I monitored Dolly closely, praying she wouldn't convulse.

My head did hit the pillow for a few minutes without interruption. I knew I would hear Dolly if she needed me. With coffee and endorphins, we made it through. I ended up working three consecutive twelve-hour shifts.

When the storm subsided, I drove for two slippery hours through a winter wonderland before stopping to pick up a pair of snowshoes from my sister-in-law. As I trudged through the remaining uneven and unploughed distance to my home, lovely white mounds of sparkling snow beckoned, enticing my fatigued brain and gritty eyelids to pause for a brief rest. It was all I could do to keep on trekking, positioning one heavy foot in front of the other. When I finally reached home, I crashed for a glorious twenty hours of unbroken sleep.

TAKE OFF ALL YOUR CLOTHES PLEASE
- ℞ - ℞ - ℞ -

Nursing is a mixed bag in this Ontario college setting, according to Judy. She loves the zoo-like quality and variety of the main campus.

ER nurses function well in this environment. All of our nurses have taken the occupational health course, and one has public health training. We've had nurses quit because they couldn't handle it. A special type of nurse is required to run a student clinic without a doctor present to make every single decision.

We get to do everything from developing educational material, to health teaching, to teaching the students on an individual basis, treating them and following up, to looking after emergencies. We also have administrative functions.

We provide information on birth control and sexually transmitted diseases (STDs), and do annual physicals because the kids are more comfortable coming here than going to their family doctors.

Recent situations that required nursing intervention include a faculty member who arrested on the tennis court, and a guest who had a stroke in the auditorium. Students have had seizures, insulin shock,

28

fractured collar bones, and have passed out with menstrual cramps.

Two nurses respond to each call to make sure we have adequate help. Two-way radios and security personnel provide good backup if we get into trouble.

Students are much more stressed than ten years ago, with everything from family, relationships, anorexia, abuse that may have happened when they were younger, and date and acquaintance rape. Everything is out in the open. Because we have two female doctors who are non-threatening and responsive, the students come to us readily.

I have this weird sense of humour that everyone has to contend with. One student complained of having a sore throat for three days. I told him the doctor would be in momentarily. As an afterthought, I added jokingly, "In the meantime, you can remove all your clothes."

The doctor couldn't believe what she saw. There he was, sitting on the chair, stark naked. He didn't realize anything was wrong. The doctor checked his throat and told him to get dressed.

"What did you tell that patient?" the doctor asked me.

"I was only kidding," I said lamely.

It's unbelievable how naive some of these kids are at college age. One girl asked if it was possible to get pregnant without having intercourse. And there's so much misinformation about the pill. We had a lot of girls this year who stopped the pill to rest their bodies. That is such a no-no, because a rest means they get pregnant and have to decide whether to continue the pregnancy or have a therapeutic abortion.

The face of our college is changing with the advent of large numbers of international students. Our college, like all colleges across Ontario, used to have enrollments of almost entirely Canadian-born students. This is no longer the case.

Many names are difficult to pronounce and we occasionally fake it with, "Mmmnnnn." On a stressful day, it doesn't take much to get us giggling.

Language is a new consideration for us. *English as a Second Language* is a popular program. International students may indicate in broken English they would like medication for a headache. We can't even give them a Tylenol until we are absolutely certain they have no allergies to medication, so we ask them to return with a translator. This can cause some difficulty, but we do have a professional responsibility not to cause them any harm. What we really need is twelve full-time interpreters in our office!

We have an expensive translator's book with basic questions in eight different languages, but the questions are too limited for our use.

Mature students have changed the focus in student health. Many students are older, while teachers are younger. I have to ask each person, "Are you staff or student? " The difference is no longer easily discernible.

Mature students expect more from the school system and from health services than the twenty-year-olds, and they come in with different illnesses. For instance, they may already have hypertension, which younger students seldom encounter. It's a whole different ball game.

Mothers and fathers who have been laid off, with anywhere up to five or more kids, are going to college while working part-time. Not only do they have the stress of learning how to study again, but they are in class with students who may be more than twenty years younger. The experience can be positive or it can be appalling.

Recently, a mature student came in crying, utterly devastated. She had drawn a blank in her final exam. After spending some time with her I learned that her oldest son was charged with armed robbery, had admitted his guilt, and was awaiting sentencing. I wrote a note suggesting she be allowed to write at a later date.

Her younger classmates neither understood nor cared. Self-centred at age twenty, they were unable to provide her with any support.

The other thing we unearthed is the incredible difference between health science students and other students. They generally are more educated before coming into the programs, have more of an understanding of health issues, and are aggressive and demanding. They don't say, "Yes Nurse," and "Thank you Nurse," they expect a detailed medical rationale.

We see naive high school kids literally bloom after three years in college and many of them keep in touch with us. It's marvellous.

A RIVETING RECITAL
- R - R - R -

As nurse Darlene found out in Labrador/Newfoundland, the whole story can't always be explained on the phone. Some things you have to see for yourself.

A lady called in saying that Valerie, her little girl, had a screw stuck in her finger, a wooden screw.

"Well, bring her up," I said.

"I can't bring her up. You'll have to get an ambulance for her."

I didn't think a little screw in the finger warranted an ambulance call.

"Surely if she has a screw in her finger, you can bring her in, can't you?"

"I can't move her," the mother explained. "She's stuck to the wood."

I called the ambulance. Valerie was a delightful little girl who had been playing outside with her brother. She was two and a half.

Down here we use a lot of Komaticks. They're like sleighs or boxes and are great to put camping gear in. Many native people use them with their dog teams, or pull them behind snowmobiles around town. In the summer the Komaticks are usually parked back of the sheds, making ideal play houses for kids and great places to keep toys.

Valerie was playing in her parents' Komatick and put her hand on a piece of wood that had a screw in it. Her brother accidentally dropped another piece of wood on top of her hand, pushing the screw right up through one of her fingers.

The ambulance attendants cut out a piece of wood — the size of an eight-by-ten picture frame — from the Komatick and brought her in, with her finger still screwed to the wood.

We couldn't get the screw out in emergency, so she went to the OR. Because the screw went through one of the joints we were concerned that she might lose the tip of her finger.

The surgery was successful and amputation was unnecessary. She stayed overnight and then returned for daily dressings. She has full function of her finger.

Every time I see her mother, she says, "You remember my little girl, she came attached to a piece of wood."

A CONSIDERABLE CHANGE
- ℞ - ℞ - ℞ -

"I'm interested in people who have suffered considerable change in their lives," says nurse Jacqueline from Ontario. "Sometimes this happens early in life, but usually it happens later."

Paul used to be a powerful vice-president in his younger days, but now, after suffering many detrimental losses in family, fortune, and health, was hospitalized with Parkinson's disease and other long-term medical problems.

He was overly aggressive and always ringing his bell. I developed a systematic strategy for responding to the bell-ringing behaviour, but I still needed to connect with him on a personal level.

One day he was lying in bed and I was sitting beside him. He was talking about Parkinson's disease. "It's like being in a coffin and having the top slammed shut," he said, "and you can't do a thing about it."

When he was in the midst of this discussion, I realized how profound it was and wanted to connect with him in any way possible. I thought of doing therapeutic touch. It was important that I not distract him, but I did want to "presence" with him.

Paul's arm was right there. I held my hand and arm just above and parallel to his. At the end of our talk he said, "I can tell you're trying to support me. It feels so good," and he made a comment about the experience of being held.

I wasn't holding him, but there was obviously such a feeling of having been attended to, that it was a powerful experience for him.

PARADOXICAL TECHNIQUES
- ℞ - ℞ - ℞ -

Nurse Alex, who works in a hyperbaric chamber unit in British Columbia, says, "This is probably different from a lot of other patient encounters, because I recently took a course in the dysfunctional section of the Family Nursing Course. *I learned about paradoxical techniques and methods of dealing with patients and wanted to try them."*

Gordon was a thirty-three-year-old single male. His diagnosis was delayed wound healing of a vascular graft, after surgical work that was done on his legs two years ago. He was diabetic.

He was slit from groin to ankle on both legs and had about two metres of incisions. Everything had healed except a small area on his right ankle. Despite dressing changes and care for the past two years, it stubbornly refused to heal.

His unemployment insurance was about to run out and, naturally, he was concerned. He couldn't work in his field as a businessman with an open wound. This was part of what he had to deal with.

He came to the hyperbaric chamber for oxygen treatments. The day he arrived we offered the usual orientation — most of our clients don't know anything about this treatment and are worried. It's also a chance for us to evaluate them, so it's a two-way street.

Gordon arrived with his girlfriend Gail, a registered nurse. They had been dating for three months. I started off with the usual greetings before getting down to business.

Gordon gave me an overview of the past two years. Intermittently Gail interrupted to add details of her own or to correct what he was saying.

"No, that's not right. This happened first, man."

They would argue a bit, but usually Gail was right, and she continued until eventually she took over the whole conversation. She was telling me about Gordon's medications, his reactions, and his activity levels.

I looked at Gordon. He was slumped in his chair, looking left out. I brought that to their attention. Indeed, Gordon said he had noticed this pattern for some time — she would take over and leave him out, especially in medical matters.

Gordon had always had a poor relationship with his father, a high-level businessman. Whenever his father and older brother, also a businessman, were conversing, they would stop in mid-sentence when Gordon entered the room, and refused to discuss business in his presence. Gordon felt his father was condescending and concentrated on his disabilities.

Running short of money from UIC, he asked his father for an allowance, who asked Gordon to draft a budget, but never had the time to review it with him. This went on for more than two months.

Consequently he had to grovel to his mother, who tried to get him to come back home. "You can't possibly live on your own," she said to her thirty-three-year-old son. She gave him small amounts of money.

This constant grovelling was very stressful. He didn't have enough money for food, and he was diabetic — he was losing sleep. He was resentful and angry, and had periods of throwing stuff around his room. "It was eating me up inside," he said.

He admitted his life was in a crisis state. He felt worthless, useless, and disempowered. He was depressed and had been on Prozac for about a year.

In order to start his hyperbaric oxygen treatments, he had to find accommodation in the area. His girlfriend suggested he come and live with her. "I'll pay your rent, provide your food, buy your medical supplies, do your dressings — you won't have to lift a finger," she promised.

Gail wanted to do everything for him, and his parents were trying to manipulate him to abide by their ways. There was so much disempowerment on Gordon's behalf. Piecing these things together, I told him he was surrounded by well-meaning people who wanted to control his life, and no one was allowing him to act on his own free will.

A bewildered Gordon agreed. I asked him what was stopping him from taking control of his own life. He said it was his leg. If he could get his leg healed, he could get on with his life.

I told him that in my opinion it was quite odd that a thirty-three-year-old, even a diabetic, would have such a problem healing a small area after he had healed so much.

I put it to him that he probably needed to have an open wound so that his father could see him as a son who wouldn't amount to anything, his mother could keep him at home for company because her husband was emotionally distant, and so his girlfriend could exercise her need to control others. I told him he was being useful to all these people.

Gail spoke first. "I agree with you." She volunteered that she was an alcoholic and had been going to AA for the last five years, and had noticed a co-dependency pattern in Gordon.

"You'd better listen to him," she said.

Gordon looked confused but remained silent. I suggested the reason for non-healing in the context that constant strain and stress produce vasoconstricting compounds in the body, which impair blood flow to the extremities. If he were to work on the emotional aspect of things, he could reduce the amount of these compounds, and initiate healing.

He agreed. He saw some value in what I said, and wanted to know what he would have to do.

"You have to look at empowering yourself," I said. Gail was supportive. "Yes, that's what you have to do."

Together, the three of us sat down to think of ways for Gordon to work toward empowerment. What we came up with was, instead of him freeloading off Gail, that he contribute financially even in a small way, help with the cooking to earn his keep, and approach Social Services. I suggested GAINS, a guaranteed annual income program for people who can't work because of disability. He said he would check to see if he qualified. I encouraged the two of them to talk about all aspects of their life. They seemed intent on being a couple and working on this problem together, and saw this as a way of helping to solidify their relationship.

When they were leaving, Gordon said, "Holy Mackerel. I came here to get an orientation for hyperbaric oxygen treatments and I'm leaving with getting my life back on track."

Two days later I got a phone call from Gail to thank me for this positive step. She said Gordon had taken it all seriously.

Gordon came in for his treatments five days later, and I noticed a difference in his persona, from the person who was dragging himself into our unit, to someone bounding with energy. He seemed like a different person. He had qualified for financial assistance, left home, and moved in with his girlfriend. He found an anonymous co-dependency support group and planned to go when Gail attended her AA meetings.

After seventeen treatments, his foot healed completely, fast for a diabetic and much less than the expected forty. I wondered how much of his recovery was due to the physical oxygen treatments, and how much was due to our discussions.

SOPHIA'S CHOICE
- ℞ - ℞ - ℞ -

"I didn't know if they were going to fire me for leaving the hospital or not," says nurse Sophia from Prince Edward Island, "but I had to go."

"I'm having terrible chest pains," Eddy said on the phone. One of our regular heart patients, he was gasping for breath at six in the morning.

His wife died the previous year, and his son usually kept watch over him.

"Is your family with you?"

"No," he said, "my son moved. He hasn't got a phone yet."

"I'll call an ambulance for you."

"The ambulance won't get here in time," he said, panic-stricken.

I handed the phone to the licensed nurses' aide (LNA) who talked to Eddy while I ran downstairs and woke the doctor up. I asked him to make a house call.

"I can't do anything for him at home," the doctor said. "Have him come in." I leapt back up the stairs.

"He dropped the phone," the LNA said.

"Call an ambulance," I said, "I'm going to get Eddy."

I grabbed some nitro and other equipment and roared off in my car.

Eddy was sitting at his kitchen table, pale and sweaty, clutching his chest. "I took a nitro but it didn't help," he said. "I feel better now that you're here."

I took his blood pressure and popped another nitro under his tongue. He was panting, his pulse irregular. I heaved him into the car.

The doctor was waiting at the ER door. We did the whole cardiac workup on Eddy, giving him IV medications to control his pain and his abnormal heartbeat. He had a heart attack, but he looked and felt much better by the time he was transferred out by ambulance.

The biggest worry of the day now that Eddy was taken care of was whether or not I going to get fired for leaving the hospital when I was the only RN on duty. Days passed and I didn't hear a thing, one way or the other.

The following week, I went to a one-day workshop on cardiac arrhythmias, a review session. I brought a copy of Eddy's EKG with me. He had gone through practically every arrhythmia in the book, and had a pacemaker put in to boot. The instructor couldn't believe it — her whole course on Eddy's single EKG.

TWO

WHEN YOUR TIME IS UP, YOUR TIME IS UP
- Я - Я - Я -

To every thing there is a season,
and a time to every purpose
under the heaven:
A time to be born,
and a time to die;

Ecclesiastes 3:1,2

Regardless of religious background, Canadian nurses give heed to the lofty wisdom of Ecclesiastes and wholeheartedly believe that when your time is up, your time is up. End of discussion.

In Greek mythology, the three Fates — Clotho, Lachesis, and Atropos, pre-date the early religions in the concept of a set time for life and death.

Each of the three white-gowned Fates had a specific duty relating to the darkness of human destiny: Clotho spun the thread of life, Lachesis fixed the length of the thread, and Atropos cut it with her shears when the span of life was done.

No one knows when Atropos will cut the thread, as the following experiences indicate. Even when a seemingly irrevocable prognosis has been made, unexplainable reversals may transpire to fulfill a preordained destiny.

Near death experiences provide fascinating accounts, but they are not all the same. Many people derive joy from positive experiences, others suffer through hellish transitions.

People who are involved in horrendous accidents may pull through despite grim predictions. Sometimes infants survive against all odds.

When Death makes its lurking presence known in the darkening shadows, its sudden emergence can catch the most prepared off guard.

At other times, the appearance of Death is foreshadowed by an incredible display of strength, grace, dignity, and love on the part of the courageous participants in Life's final drama.

THE OPERATING ROOM LIST
- ℞ - ℞ - ℞ -

A miracle is a marvellous event due to a supernatural agency. Virginia, one of the 8,424 nurses in New Brunswick, encountered a miracle without even looking for one.

One of my assignments on evenings was to prepare a surgical patient, Mrs. Eclaire, for a total bowel resection for the following morning. She was seventy-five years old.

She had a large tumour in her bowel and was fairly obstructed as a result. The surgeons decided to remove as much as they could, and do a colostomy.

Mrs. Eclaire was my surgical case study for a presentation I was making, so I had researched all her reports in detail and examined her x-rays. The tumour was well documented and I had been able to palpate it easily myself.

I explained what I was going to do for her, in preparation for the OR — the whole nine yards, with preps and enemas.

"That's lovely dearie," she said. "You need someone to practice on, but I'm not going to the operating room tomorrow."

I thought, with my luck, they probably had cancelled her. I checked with the charge nurse. No cancellations, she was still booked.

"According to the operating room list," I said, "you're booked for ten tomorrow morning."

After I completed the pre-operative procedures, she said, "I know I'm on your list dearie, but I'm not going to have an operation tomorrow. I won't need it."

The next afternoon I was psyched up to look after my fresh post-op bowel resection, but Mrs. Eclair was sitting in a chair, getting ready to go home.

The doctors had made grand surgical rounds in the morning, before she was booked for the OR. Numerous interns and residents came in to palpate her abdomen, but they couldn't feel anything.

They thought this strange and sent her down to x-ray for a flat plate of her abdomen. Nothing. They did a barium enema. Nothing. The tumour was gone.

"I knew I wouldn't have an operation, dearie," she said to me. "I knew I was going to be healed before I went to your operating room."

She felt her healing was a gift from God. Devout and religious, she had prayed for a healing, as had her church. To her there was no question it would happen.

I wasn't skeptical, because if there's anything I can say today after twenty-five years in this business, it's that a lot more happens that's unexplained, than is explained.

Lillian R. Tymchuk, RN

TWENTY MINUTES TO LIVE
- ℞ - ℞ - ℞ -

"I've always said nursing is a profession you have to love, or you can't do it," says Julie, a sharp emergency room nurse in Saskatchewan. "I truly believe that."

She has no doubt that excelling in this profession takes its toll, particularly in the gray area bridging consciousness and unconsciousness.

Motorcycle accident. Ran off the road and into a telephone pole that literally sliced him in two. The pole broke through his pelvis and perineum and came up through his hip.

The ambulance drivers stuffed a jacket into his abdominal cavity to hold his guts in, and strapped his legs together to create some pressure. When they brought him in, he was fully conscious.

Nothing could be done. He had ruptured his bladder and torn his bowel in a thousand places. We started IVs and other measures we knew weren't going to help. The only thing we could do really was watch him bleed to death. It took twenty minutes.

He was twenty-three. On his way home from visiting his wife and infant son in the hospital. The happiest man in the world. All of a sudden — BOOM.

The injuries were in his lower body. No head injury. We gave him medication for pain. Didn't touch him.

"There's absolutely nothing we can do for you," the doctor said. "If you have something to say, say it now."

In that twenty minutes, it was like a revealing of all the nasty things he had ever done to his mother and father, and the fact that he wouldn't see his infant son grow up. "Tell my wife I love her," he pleaded.

Talk about a heartbreaker. One of the worst single accidents I've ever seen, physically and emotionally. I dreamt about it for a long time.

Every time we have a bad trauma, I go to bed knowing I'll dream about it. And every time we have a code, I wake up in the middle of the night, running the code. It's something I live with.

THE WIDE-BRIMMED HAT
- R - R - R -

The expression "out of sight, out of mind" has no place in Lucy's professional nursing practice in Quebec. The care and concern she shows her patients go far beyond any institutional walls.

In outpatient oncology, patients on chemotherapy received a certain amount of teaching, precautions, and an overall "what to do." At the same time, as nurses we tried to complete a psycho-social assessment, knowing how terrible cancer can be on one's life and all it affects.

I looked after Justine, an artist who had developed breast cancer. A determined lady, she had stopped treatment at another hospital, and came here to see our doctors.

Her chemotherapy had already started and she always wore a beautiful, big-brimmed, black velvet hat because she was too proud to wear a wig. That I found out later.

Justine would sit in front of me while I was doing her treatment, and listened, but she wouldn't look at me. The brim of her hat was at eye level, so I had a hard time monitoring any reaction. Was she listening to me? What was her facial expression?

Needless to say, on that first occasion I didn't phrase any personal questions or try to do a more exact assessment of her life situation. But I tried to stay with her each time she came in for treatment. Slowly she started to talk and I sensed the formation of a bond.

She started to feel confident enough to open up a bit more. She told me how annoyed she was about the manner in which she was approached at the other hospital. There were too many questions which she felt invaded her privacy. These were questions I also normally asked.

But slowly she did talk to me. I didn't ask questions. I would rephrase what she said and she would provide more information. I found out she was a single mother with a fifteen-year-old daughter named Clarette. The teenager had a lot of trouble coping with her mother's disease.

Justine tried to reorganize her life, but the many side effects of her chemotherapy made that difficult. At one point she brought Clarette with her to the clinic, and the two agreed to see the social worker.

In this way we were able to link them to a support group. Justine agreed, wanting to ensure a family approach to the whole process. I was happy with that, because at first I never thought it would be possible.

She was with us almost two years, but she didn't respond to the chemotherapy and deteriorated. When she was admitted to the palliative care unit I followed up on her. Clarette and I had become close enough that she, too, welcomed my visits. I saw Justine a lot less but, from the nursing point of view, I was caring for more than a patient, even if I wasn't providing direct care anymore.

She became confused when the cancer metastasized to the brain, and she died soon thereafter. I valued meeting and knowing her. I thought it rewarding, as a nurse, to have the opportunity to develop such a relationship with a patient and family, to apply nursing theories, and to see that sometimes they do work.

THE GOOD DIE EARLY
- ℞ - ℞ - ℞ -

Tina, an experienced emergency room nurse in Saskatchewan, shares a compelling experience embodying the fascinating approach of the Three Fates.

Despite all the latest medical technology to assist in providing an accurate prognosis, the information proved to be wrong. "I was afraid my patient would be dead before morning," Tina says.

Late Sunday afternoon a hillbilly-type garbed in torn coveralls, muddied boots, and an old hat, trudged in with a younger parody of himself. Pierce was Elton's grandson.

Elton was upset. He had driven here in his pick-me-up truck from the country, he said, because they sent him to get some "thing" for his neck.

"First, I need to ask you what happened," I said.

Pierce had been driving the pick-me-up and rolled it in some field. They crawled out, got into a different pick-me-up, and drove to a rural hospital.

Elton said his neck hurt, but the hospital wanted to charge thirty dollars for "this piece of collar" to go around his neck. He refused to pay, so he trundled on into the city. Pierce was not hurt.

"Maybe we better check you out and make sure everything's okay," I suggested. I was concerned he might have a fracture, and wanted to stabilize his neck. I tried to put a collar on him, but he wouldn't have any part of it. "How be I just wrap a towel around your neck to hold it steady?"

He could live with that, so I taped a towel in place, and asked his grandson to push him to x-ray in a wheelchair.

"Don't take that towel off no matter what," I warned, wagging my forefinger in his face for extra emphasis. He smiled. When they didn't return for a while, I went to x-ray, looking for them.

Pierce was sitting in the wheelchair, happily rolling himself back and forth and singing, while his grandpa was in the bathroom. When Elton re-appeared, the towel was off. The x-ray tech was flying around, screaming his head off. How dare I send a patient over there in a wheelchair and a towel, instead of a stretcher and a Philadelphia collar? I yelled back.

But Elton had broken his neck, high up on his cervical spine. He was a tall, heavy man — not heavy fat, but heavy big. One wrong move and he'd be paralyzed for life.

In the meantime, Elton figured he was on his way out the door because he had his x-ray. The x-ray tech and I were going nuts trying to get Elton and Pierce to come back to ER. I finally convinced them, and called the neurosurgeon on call.

We had to convince Elton that he needed immediate treatment in the form of halo traction, and we needed his consent to treatment. We encouraged him to remove those clothes of his and change into a hospital gown.

The ER physician wanted to put Gardiner tongs on him because that was the treatment of choice at the moment, and it was fast. But no way was anybody going to stick pins in his head, said Elton.

Then the doctor decided on a strykker frame — it sandwiches the patient between two heavy canvas sheets and stabilizes him, while it can be rotated to change the position of the patient. Elton's feet hung way over the edge of the canvas, making for an unbelievable scenario.

In the meantime, the neurosurgeon was one of those doctors who was trying to teach his two little boys the realities of life. If he had a patient in ICU, for example, he would have the boys come in and watch while they pulled the plug on somebody. We shuddered at the thought.

He brought them in to help put the halo on. They were six and eight, much too young to be anywhere near patients, let alone in ER. My nerves were shattered by this time.

"No, you're not going to have the boys help you," I yelled. I chased them out of the room. "Go and sit in the front office and WAIT," I screamed.

We got the halo on Elton. Pierce didn't have a sniff of a clue what was going on. While he continued to roll himself back and forth in the wheelchair, I told him what a wonderful thing he had done by driving his grandpa in, that now his grandpa had to be admitted to the hospital for surgery, and how lucky his grandpa was to be alive. We tried to get him to realize how critical the situation was, to no avail.

Elton was sandwiched on the strykker frame, the halo was in place, but we had no jacket big enough to fit him. It's a front-to-back plastic jacket that goes with the halo. Bars slide into it and connect to the halo to keep it stable. Without the jacket, the halo is a ring around the head that serves no purpose. We had to send to Toronto to get a jacket big enough to fit him.

So I'm thinking, this is a dead man. There's no way he could survive till morning. The surgeons wanted to operate, to do a fusion first thing in the morning, but Elton refused surgery. He remained unyielding in his position.

Three weeks later Elton walked out of the hospital, perfectly healthy and happy. He had no deficits — nothing. He didn't have a clue how seriously he had been injured.

It renewed my faith in fate. I say when it's your time, it's going to happen, and when it isn't your time, forget it. And this is the perfect example.

THE TRIANGLE
- ₽ - ₽ - ₽ -

"I had a ruptured cerebral aneurysm, but I'm just too mean to die." This is how Ontario medical nurse Joyce initiates her fascinating report.

An excruciating headache didn't stop me from working. Being a nurse, I diagnosed myself. I'd had headaches before and thought Holy Toledo, now I'm a migraine sufferer.

I was sent home where I collapsed in the bathroom, without any idea what had hit me. I was taken to hospital, and the following day, had surgery. An aneurysm ruptured in the right mid-cerebral area, and the neurosurgeon went in behind my right eye, leaving that area radically swollen and painful.

I don't know when this next experience occurred, but I must have been on the respirator because I couldn't move my head. It was pitch black, like being in dense woods in the country, with no sunshine and no stars.

To the right, in my peripheral vision, I could see a bright triangle of light. The game was to look at it, because if I took my eyes from it, it moved closer — and I thought I would die if it touched me.

I played the game until I became so tired that I fell asleep, but it was very real and frightening to me. I was fighting for my life. After the initial surgery, I had to be rushed to the OR once more to have a drain inserted. I was deathly afraid, and my right eye was killing me.

However, the days passed and my condition gradually improved. With the help of my family and friends and a lot of painstaking therapy, I recovered fully. I had always been terrible with names before my surgery, and that remained the case afterward.

After taking a year off I went back to work, this time in palliative care. But I always carried the picture of the triangle with me. I couldn't understand — why a triangle?

Over time I became aware of my husband's involvement with another woman, and we separated two years after my surgery. I now had an interpretation for the triangle — me, my husband, and his girlfriend.

At work, a tall Englishman by the name of Arthur was one of my patients. He had a malignant brain tumour, an astrocytoma. He had completed a course of chemotherapy following surgery which did not completely remove the tumour.

His wife and son were coming to see him on the weekend, so I suggested he stay up a bit longer each day so he could sit up for their entire visit. "That'll be a nice surprise for them, don't you think?"

"Yes," he said. I could see he was pleased.

Another nurse and I sat him on the side of the bed and pivoted him into the chair. Nurses really have to bench press 3,000 pounds just to do their work. I was on my knees putting his slippers on when he passed out. I thought, he's going to die in this chair.

He came to and I asked him what happened.

"I don't know," he said. "I'm so weak."

The next day he looked too pale to attempt getting him out of bed. As I reached for a basin he passed out again.

"Arthur, what's happening to you, Arthur?"

"Oooohhh, okay ... okay."

"You all right?"

"I feel weak."

He passed out again.

"Johnny, Johnny." Then, I realized that I was calling him by the wrong name. No wonder he wasn't responding.

"Arthur. What's happening to you?"

"I'm dying."

"I know you are, Arthur. What's it like?"

"Really dark."

"You've got to tell me about this, Arthur." I told him about my experience with the triangle.

"Did it ever touch you?" he asked.

"No."

"That's good. Because I saw it too."

And then it hit me ... the triangle was Father, Son, and Holy Ghost. Two days later, Arthur's time came and he died. After our insightful discussion, I thought the religious aspect of the triangle more likely, and that was comforting to me.

WHERE THERE'S SMOKE
- ᴙ - ᴙ - ᴙ -

Nadia, an outpost nurse in northern Saskatchewan, claims that the relentless role fate plays in our lives was strongly reinforced by one of her patients. "This lady will continue to deny that she smokes to her dying day," she says.

Fanny was an eighty-five-year-old lady who lived in her own home with her alcoholic nephew, Bill. Always impaired, he remained friendly and soft-spoken.

He made sure she got up in the mornings, prepared her meals, and did everything in his limited power to ease her plight.

Fanny was a sweetheart with cardiac, respiratory, and every other imaginable medical problem. Despite all this, she refused to give up smoking. Her fingers revealed the dirty, yellow-brown colour of chronic smokers, but she denied smoking. "Bill smokes," she'd say with a twinkle in her eye, "but I don't."

Her most serious problem was loneliness. She wanted to live in the nursing home where her friends were, but couldn't get past the long waiting list.

She called me two or three times a day and I found that going to see her each time wasn't such a big deal. Her house was early third-world country, and she lived mostly in her bedroom. As we chatted, her vague complaints dissipated into thin air. She was on continuous humidified oxygen, and the green oxygen tank in her living room surely had enough tubing to reach the coast of Newfoundland.

"No smoking in the house, Fanny. You or Bill. Remember." I gave her the same warning every day.

We settled into a routine that she was comfortable with. Faithfully she called me in the morning and in the late evening. I told her I would be there, and I was. Then I didn't have to worry about her calling me at three or four in the morning.

Needless to say, she got neglected the odd time, when I got too busy with other patients. And sometimes I did forget about her. She punished me for this breach by calling in the middle of the night, saying she needed to see me immediately, for one phoney reason or another.

The time came when I was preparing to go home to southern Saskatchewan for my holidays. I finished eight hours in the clinic and was on call for the next twelve. Fanny called that evening, and I put her to bed as usual.

I was tired and needed my sleep. At three in the morning my phone rang. It was Fanny.

"Nadia, you must come."

"I was just there, Fanny. I'll see you in the morning, before I leave."

"You have to come. I'm on fire."

"That's a good one, Fanny, but you mustn't do that."

She had called wolf so many times, and I thought Fanny figured this was really funny.

"No, seriously. I'm on fire."

"Fanny, I'll see you at seven in the morning — and that's probably the best one I've ever heard. Okay?"

Bill got on the line, his words slurred. "This woman, she's on fire. I threw water on her." And he hung up.

I decided I'd better check this one out. I drove to her house and opened the screen door. I could smell singed chicken.

Fanny was sitting on her bed, sopping wet, hair spiked up like a cone man. Her eyelashes, eyebrows, and the hair in her nose were all gone. Her face was black.

Charcoal, really. All I could see were smoke-stained teeth and the whites of her eyes — actually her eyes were like cantaloupes because the fire had followed the path of the oxygen tubing and went up her nose. Her feet were black as black could be.

"Fanny, how are you?"

"I'm fine," she said. She looked like a one-hundred-and-ninety-year-old drowned rat. Her nephew had poured water all over her and went back to bed, leaving a good two inches of water on the bedroom floor. He saw no reason to stay up.

It was like a science fiction movie. I wanted to phone the RCMP to come and take pictures, but they would have killed me. Why the entire house didn't blow up was a mystery. And there, in the ashtray beside her bed, were thirty thousand lipstick-stained cigarette butts.

"Smoking a little, Fanny?"

"I don't smoke, Nadia. It's Bill what does."

She had second and third degree burns and smoke inhalation. It would have taken too long to get an air ambulance, so I drove her the fifty miles to the hospital in my car.

Fanny was something else. She told the nurses there that she must have lit a cigarette in her sleep, because she certainly didn't smoke when she was awake. She was air-vacced to a burn unit down south. How she survived despite ensuing infections, I'll never know.

DADDY, DON'T DIE
- R - R - R -

"I did not anticipate a miracle," documents nurse *Alice from Alberta. "My patient was uremic and dying."*

At two in the morning, I didn't expect Jerry to last till dawn. He had refused dialysis and now lay comatosed. In checking his chart, I realized he was Roman Catholic and hadn't had the Last Rites performed. I called the priest, who came in quickly.

The next time I looked in on Jerry, he was sitting up in bed, but he looked agitated as I approached. "Get away from me," he screeched. "Don't come near me."

His eyes dilated, terrified.

"It's okay, Jerry," I said gently.

"Don't touch me. Stay away."

He eventually settled down and fell asleep.

The following day I left for a two-week holiday. When I returned he was still alive, much to my surprise.

"You," he said, pointing a bony finger at me. "I remember you. You were in my room when I was so ill."

"Yes I was," I acknowledged.

"I thought I was dead and had gone to heaven. In my mind, you were an angel but I was terrified of you. Then, through a dense kind of fog, I heard my little girl saying, 'Daddy, don't die. I need you. When are you coming home?'"

In that strange, semi-conscious state, he decided to accept treatment. He went on dialysis, got a transplant, and lived to watch his happy little girl grow up.

THE BIG BLACK BOOK
- ₽ - ₽ - ₽ -

In Ontario, nurse Marlene discovered that the love and concern some relatives show their loved ones is something that can't be taught.

I'm five feet one inch and Molly was shorter, making me feel tall for a change. Her husband of sixty years, Al, had congestive heart failure and pneumonia. When he developed emphysema, she attended classes held in the hospital to find out what he had to contend with. Both were in their early eighties.

She showed up every day, rain or shine, love shining through her cataract-clouded eyes. It was obvious there was nothing she wouldn't do for him.

He ended up on our cancer floor because there were no other beds available, and he became our pet. We got him strong enough to go home, but several months later, he again developed pneumonia and was admitted to the ICU. Within days he was able to leave ICU, and he asked to return to our floor. It was like coming home for him.

"I'm glad you're here," I told him. "We'll concentrate on getting you well."

We got him settled into his old bed, all smiles and happy. As usual, his loving Molly was at his side. She watched while he dozed. When he woke up, he told her to go home and get some rest.

"Okay, my darling," she replied. "I'll be back after supper."

"Good-bye, my love," he said. His eyes never left her until she disappeared from view.

As soon as Molly got home she had the strongest urge to return. But before she could turn around, the phone rang. It was the hospital. Al had died.

A lot of these patients wait until their loved ones go home, and then they die. I also think Al waited to die until he came back to our floor, because we all cared about him so much.

I truly believe there is a Big Black Book up there that says you're going to die on such and such a day, at such and such a time. You never go before your time.

I've seen it too often, where people have been so low and I think they're going to be gone in a couple of hours and they aren't. They wait and wait — for what? And then boom, they die. It's uncanny.

Another patient had a wife who absolutely adored him. He had primary cancer in the nostril, and had Commando surgery. This is major surgery involving the nose, cheekbones, and jaw. His face was one big cavity.

After the surgery, his wife bought a trailer and took him camping outdoors, something he always loved to do. How many people would take a spouse home in that condition and look after him? She told me she used to put raw steak on his face and the cancer would eat it — that's something I've never seen.

When he had to be hospitalized again, all he had was his forehead, his eyes, and his false teeth. You could see the cancer eating away at the little sacs under his eyes. I said to the doctor, "I hope he dies before his eyes fall out, because that would really make me sick."

He was on Morphine tablets for pain, which was fine when he had his teeth in, and we knew approximately where to put the pills. If he took his teeth out, it was bad news.

Still mentally alert, he watched me for any reaction to his appearance. I had to walk in as though he was normal-looking.

We usually used IV Morphine and Dilaudid for more effective pain control, but his wife was afraid an IV would prolong his life. "He needs the IV for pain control," I explained. "This is not going to prolong his life."

Finally I convinced her, and we gradually increased his medication so he wouldn't suffer. Despite megadoses of Morphine, he remained aware of his surroundings.

He started getting anxious, as many terminal patients do, so we gave him Valium to relax. He could no longer speak verbally, but his eyes spoke volumes. One evening he quietly passed away.

We've had patients with tumours on their neck that started out as little red dots. One patient had a tumour that had grown to the point where it pushed his head in the opposite direction. It was extremely sad, but we have to treat these people with the dignity they deserve until their time comes.

TRUE LOVE
- ℞ - ℞ - ℞ -

For Grace, nursing part-time in Alberta is perfect, and her profession fills a deep-seated need for her.

"I feel nurses are privileged to be at their patients' side when they give birth and when they die," she says.

What's so special about being a nurse in a small town is knowing most of the people, stopping on the street to say hello, and becoming a part of their lives.

Andrew and Helen were two of these people. He was seventy-four and she was eight years his junior. She had never married until she met him in her fifties. They were so neat, always walking hand-in-hand. I enjoyed their company and spent quite a bit of time with them.

After ten happy years of marriage he was diagnosed with cancer, and for the last year was in and out of hospital. When it was apparent that he was terminal, we allowed her to stay overnight. That's the way it works in a small hospital — we try to accommodate people.

One night he wasn't doing well and she wasn't able to sleep either. She kept going in and out of his room. We weren't busy so I said, "Let's have a cup of tea and we'll go and sit with him."

She knew the end was coming. For an hour, she and I sat together and talked at his bedside. She told me about her husband and how wonderful their life together was. All the time she was holding his hand. It was therapeutic for both of them and there was lots of touching.

During that magical interval, we both cried. I had known her for a long time and we had that special bond. It was good to be there, to be able to support her through this. After we finished our tea she said, "I think I'll go back to bed now. I feel okay."

I sat beside her for a while after she went to bed. Later, she got up and returned to his room, and he died shortly after. I gave her a big hug.

Afterward Helen sent me a heartwarming card expressing her gratitude that I was her husband's nurse when his time came.

Lillian R. Tymchuk, RN

TWO MIRACLES
- ℞ - ℞ - ℞ -

"I've seen two miracles in my life," reports nurse Nancy from the Yukon. "The first one was professional and sent me on a quest for God. The second one was personal and, for me, confirmed the presence of God."

Mrs. McDonald was diagnosed with abdominal cancer, but the diagnosis came too late. She was in the end stages, no longer conscious or responsive. She had an intravenous running but other than that, her family was waiting for her to die. She hadn't had anything to eat or drink for days.

I was working an evening shift when some of her friends came in and prayed with the family. When the call light went on, I thought that's it, they're calling to say she died.

But when I went in to the room, she was sitting up in bed and asked me for a cup of tea. I was stunned.

From there, she got better and went home. The doctors couldn't figure out why it had happened because she was moribund, waiting for death. I certainly didn't know why she got better. It obviously wasn't her time to go, but I thought it was a miracle. There was no other explanation.

This experience awakened something in me. It made me question where this miracle could have come from. Did God really do it? I wondered how much in control we really are. It was a good experience for me, because I used to think if we couldn't do something, no one could.

I started looking for Whoever, that Greater Being. I went to different churches and talked to all kinds of people. I started my own personal quest.

Since then I've had children of my own, and my oldest child had Legge-Perthes disease. I didn't know what it was until she got it. It's a necrotic head of the femur, and in her case, it also involved the growth plate. The course of the disease progressed from the time she was seven until she was eleven. The disease left her right leg shorter than her left one.

Because she had a limp, I took her to a physiotherapist to see if she could get a lift for her shoes. I was worried about the alignment in her back. He wasn't sure how to go about it and referred us to an orthopedic surgeon. So we went south to Alberta.

The surgeon measured her legs and said she required corrective surgery. He could either make her left leg shorter or the right one longer, but probably he would lengthen the right one.

I knew the power of prayer and my daughter had been prayed for at different times. When we went back to see the surgeon in six months time, he kept measuring her leg over and over. "Her leg is no different," he said. "It's exactly the same as the other one. I don't understand it."

"Thank God, He did it."

"He must have," he said, "because I don't have any other explanation for it. Her right leg was definitely shorter before but now she's okay. I don't need to operate."

It wasn't like ZAP — her leg got longer. Or maybe it was, I don't know. I didn't realize her legs were the same length until the surgeon measured them. Somewhere within that six month period, her right leg grew in.

She's thirteen now and just went on the Chilkoot Climb, a thirty-seven-mile mountain climbing experience. They climb 3,700 feet up the Chilkoot Mountain Pass where the gold miners scrambled during the goldrush. It's an historical climb that people in this area like to complete. She carried a twenty-five-pound pack and had no difficulty.

This puts the pieces back in the puzzle — I now know that the first miracle was Him. Dedicating my life to God has made all the difference.

I always thought if God was really God, then it had to be more than a one hour session on a Sunday morning, like it used to be for me. After I found out how much more there is, I felt He came home with me after church and became part of my daily life. He gives me hope and an inner peacefulness. I think it has made me more compassionate toward people when I see their plight.

It's also made me a better nurse. I've had several patients whom I've talked to about God, when they asked me to, and some whom I've prayed for, and it's given them comfort. Personally, I derive a lot of consolation from knowing that God is with me always.

A TRIP TO THE MALL
- R - R - R -

An Alberta hospice. A "routine" night with a "routine" death. The next night, however, nurse Rachel did not get off quite so easily.

I was working by myself with six patients, and my first night was typical. I did have a woman die in the morning, but it was pretty straightforward. She was an older lady and her son was with her. Her death was peaceful. Because she died at the end of my shift, another nurse took over.

The next night when I came on I went around and checked everybody as usual. Sandy, a young woman whom I had admitted previously, was thirty-two and diagnosed with cancer of the lung. The door to her room was shut.

I was told by the evening nurse that her husband Richard was with her, and that they had requested some privacy. As a rule we don't go in if there's family present. Even if they are there for four hours, we leave them alone. Of course, we get to know the family a bit first, and make sure there's no funny business going on.

After making rounds, I returned to the desk and did some of the night work, filling out requisitions and filing charts. I was a bit nervous about being there alone at night.

I heard someone running and hoped it was only the resident attendant who looked after the pre-hospice

69

people. The hospice used to be a seniors' lodge at one time, and several seniors still lived there. But it was Richard.

"I think my wife passed away," he said.

I walked back with him to the room. Her bed was empty as was the pullout couch. I kept thinking how much I wished I wasn't there.

"Where is she?" I asked.

"Over there," he said, pointing.

She was on the floor. Dead. It's hard to describe, but she was on her bent knees, and her face was flat on the floor with her arms behind her. On the way down, she had hit a beautiful arrangement of dried flowers that Richard's office had sent, and the flowers stuck grotesquely out of her mouth.

I was taken aback and wondered what best to do. I was the only one there, plus this resident attendant, but she was on the other side of the building.

Everything seemed unreal. In in-service classes, we were reminded over and over that this was a hospice, not a hospital. If we were at home, what would we do? That's what we were told to always remember.

I thought if I were at home, I would fix her up. I asked him if he wanted me to put her on the bed.

"Do you have to?" he asked quietly.

"No, I don't," I replied, breathing a sigh of relief. I wondered how I possibly could have done that anyway. I removed the flowers and changed her position so that she looked half decent, as though she were lying in bed. I placed her head on a pillow, and covered her up.

Richard told me they had been cuddling in bed when she said she had to go to the bathroom. He got her sitting up on the side of the bed, and then went to get the commode. Sandy had little space left in her lungs, and her respirations and colour left a lot to be desired. By the time he returned with the commode, she had slid off the bed — and that was it.

Given the setting, it was intimate and horrendous at the same time. I reassembled the pullout couch and he and I sat and talked about their life together and their children. We talked about her illness and how the children had only known a sick mother, and the fact that Sandy had never been close to her own family, although they had been in to see her earlier that day. He had a strong faith and prayed out loud. He accepted that her time had come.

He was calm, cool, and collected. I don't know where he got his strength. I suppose he may have said the same about me, but I felt like I was going to die. I couldn't believe this had happened, even though I knew her death was imminent. With cancer of the lung, though, you never know.

Later, I removed her jewellery, gave it to Richard, and left him while I phoned the doctor who asked to speak to "the husband."

Richard's voice seemed to echo in the deathly silence of the hospice, but a hospice can make quiet seem loud. I tried to escape his voice but couldn't. He commended the doctor for everything he had done for his wife. I couldn't believe anyone could feel that way about a doctor at such a time, and was surprised how much he praised him.

I went to the funeral. I didn't know if I should have gone or not, but after the church service, Richard mouthed a silent "thank you" to me.

A year later I saw him at the mall, but I couldn't make myself speak to him. I couldn't go up to him and say, "I'm the nurse who was with your wife the night she died."

If the setting had been different — something more private than a mall — perhaps I would have. Then both of us would have had a chance to handle the many turbulent feelings and emotions that were guaranteed to resurface.

THE GOOD SAMARITAN
- R - R - R -

The Good Samaritan found a man half dead and "bound up his wounds, pouring in oil and wine, and set him on his own beast, and brought him to an inn, and took care of him."

The following clinical account from nurse Sarah in Prince Edward Island closely parallels the Biblical parable.

At 4:20 A.M. an eighteen-year-old male was brought into the hospital by a good samaritan. Actually it was a fisherman on his way to work who found him in the middle of the road lying in a pool of blood. The fisherman remained to offer his assistance.

On arrival the patient was bleeding profusely and in cardiogenic shock. He had two large lacerations on his occiput and a flap laceration under which his skull was clearly depressed.

He had a swollen right shoulder with marked bruising over the other shoulder. Over his back was a generalized contusion as though he had been dragged over a hard surface. He had a large wound on his left leg which was spurting blood. The patient was confused and uncooperative and was throwing himself around.

With the help of the good samaritan holding him, the licensed nurses' aide grabbed an abdominal pad, and put her hand in the wound to stop the bleeding. An IV was started immediately to run wide open and pressure bandages were applied to the bleeding points. The pupils were equal and reactive to light.

The patient's condition became progressively worse and I took the time out to call a second RN in for help. She lived a couple of minutes away at the bottom of the hill.

The immediate assessment revealed the injuries were inflicted by a hit-and-run car accident. Several sutures were inserted to control the bleeding as soon as the doctor arrived. The patient was then transferred to our county hospital via ambulance, escorted by the doctor on call.

There he had a subclavian line inserted and three other IVs. He had x-rays of the skull, chest, and abdomen done. Blood was drawn for serum alcohol. The patient was then transferred to the major centre. There he had an emergency laparotomy and splenectomy done for a ruptured spleen.

He was subsequently transferred to New Brunswick for further evaluation of his head injuries. About a month later he came back here to convalesce. It wasn't his time to go.

SUDDEN DEATH
- R - R - R -

Emergency room nurse Violet has seen practically every possible reaction to sudden death in Saskatchewan. Practically.

At a civic function in honour of Thanksgiving, the guest speaker got up and started his speech. A few minutes into it he asked for a glass of water. Somebody rushed right up with one and never thought anything about it. The next thing anyone knew, the speaker was slumped behind the podium.

Everyone thought he must have dropped a paper. When he didn't get up for a while, the master of ceremonies checked him. He had arrested.

After the initial confusion somebody started CPR. They brought him to the hospital and we worked on him for about half an hour, but it was too late. He was dead.

The interesting part of this was not the fact that the man had arrested, but the reaction of all the people. There must have been at least fifteen cars that pulled up to ER, and people stood outside, waiting to see what was going to happen. That fascinated me. Someone had gone to find his wife, and while I was waiting for her to come, more people came to stand and stare.

When the wife arrived I took her into the office and was waiting for the doctor to come and talk to her. Of course, she knew immediately what must have happened to her husband. I said we were sorry. She went absolutely bananas and started to beat me up. She couldn't accept her husband's fate.

"It's your fault. What did you do?" she screamed at the top of her lungs. "You didn't try hard enough. How dare you do this to my husband?"

Talk about an uncomfortable situation. I knew she wasn't in control of herself and yet I wondered where this reaction came from. A state of denial is certainly common and even expected among family members and loved ones who are dealing with sudden death or any type of unexpected trauma, but still, it makes you wonder, really and truly.

Lillian R. Tymchuk, RN

JUST A PIECE OF ICE, MORE OR LESS
- R - R - R -

"He was frozen solid when we got him. There was no heart beat, no blood pressure, no nothing. He was just a piece of ice, more or less."

With such an initial picture, the last thing Newfoundland/Labrador emergency room nurse Carol expected was a miraculous recovery.

He had been out in the snow all night and it was minus fifty degrees with the windchill factor. The RCMP found him at eight in the morning and brought him to our ER. We went to work on him.

First we warmed him up, of course, while doing CPR. We started at the core of the body by putting a gastric lavage tube into his stomach, and a urethral catheter into his bladder. We continually flushed warm water through these tubes. We warmed his abdomen by peritoneal dialysis.

We don't have a microwave, so we had to pour scorching hot water into a big sink to warm up the IVs and other fluids. One nurse looked after this task exclusively.

We were kept going. There was one nurse for the gastric lavage, one for the peritoneal dialysis, and one for the urethral catheter. We did this for four hours straight. We didn't worry too much about his extremities because we figured they were pretty well gone anyway.

At twelve noon we got a pulse. It was miraculous because when he came in, his temperature wasn't registering on the low grade rectal probe that reads down to twenty-two degrees Celsius.

We couldn't smell any alcohol and when we did the analysis of his stomach contents in our lab there was no alcohol content. But later, the RCMP said that alcohol was involved. I don't know where they got that from, but they had reason to believe he was drunk.

Once we got him stabilized we flew him out to a major centre for further treatment. Despite partial amputations of his extremities, he survived and returned home. Under the circumstances, his was a miraculous recovery.

THE POWER OF PRAYER
- R - R - R -

"We get lots of really bad trauma and many serious head injuries. But I've seen first-hand the power of prayer in the most dramatic cases," says ICU nurse Sheila in Saskatchewan.

We received one young trauma victim who had totally enucleated the right side of his brain in a serious car accident.

He was found hanging upside down in the car, and the only reason he survived in the first place was because his head was tilted back in a way that kept his

77

airway open. The other kids who were with him were killed instantly.

They were going to make him an organ donor, but for some reason he kept on living. His parents and whole family prayed over him every day.

In three weeks, he was out of intensive care, absolutely aware of everything that was going on. He walked out of the hospital with no deficits, perfectly healthy.

We attribute part of his recovery to his family's prayers. And it just wasn't his time to go.

AGAINST ALL ODDS
- Ŗ - Ŗ - Ŗ -

"She wasn't supposed to be here," muses nursery nurse Maureen in Manitoba. "To all of us, she was a miracle baby."

This baby was transported to our nursery from another hospital. She had barely rolled through the doors of our nursery when she went flat so we immediately went into action.

She had a blood vessel that ruptured and she actually lost four times her body volume in blood, and required transfusions. Before she was twenty-four hours old she suffered severe asphyxia and arrested three times. Needless to say, everybody was concerned about her neurological status and the doctors spoke to her parents.

This family had great faith in God, and kept telling us the baby was going to be okay, and that they could accept whatever happened to her as long as we did everything possible to help her.

While she still is not out of the woods, she looks around and smiles at her mom and dad, and does everything she's supposed to be doing. Had you laid odds, no one who was there that first night ever thought she could survive. At the very least, we thought she would have brain damage. We started IVs and transfused her while keeping her tiny little airway patent. The doctors went in and clamped the ruptured blood vessel and repaired the damage to the surrounding tissues — right there in the middle of the nursery. During this critical surgery she arrested, necessitating CPR and life-saving drugs.

Yet here's this little one who's looking around and taking her feeds and breathing on her own and doing things that babies do. Her parents are so thankful for all the care she received, for the nurses, and for the prayers.

They feel the prayers of their small group of friends and their community helped her to survive, along with the care we provided.

THREE

FROM THE NURSE'S POINT OF VIEW
- R - R - R -

A faithful friend is the medicine of life.

Ecclesiasticus 6:16

Canadian nurses encounter joys and tribulations in both their professional and personal lives, learning something of value from each new experience that life has to offer.

There are times when the personal point of view of the nurse automatically intertwines with her professional work. For example, an unidentified gentleman in his late forties was rushed into one of Ontario's busy emergency departments amid wailing sirens and flashing lights. He was in full cardiac arrest. Despite the best of care, the gentleman died.

One of the nurses reached into his pocket to look for identification. Instead of finding a wallet, however, she pulled out a love letter written by a lady other than his wife.

All belongings are normally given to the family upon their arrival, but this nurse could not see adding to the wife's grief. Without a moment's hesitation she ripped the love letter into countless shreds. As she pitched the last bit into the garbage can, in strode the Coroner.

"What's this?" he demanded angrily. He insisted she tape the letter back to its original form. After reading it, he instructed one of the police officers to go to the lady's home to inform her of her lover's death.

"Tell her not to write any more letters," he said.

In the meantime, the gentleman's wife and children came in, delayed by city traffic. They were notified of the death of their loving husband and father.

Nurses deal with personal and professional challenges, each in her own particular way. In the diversity of stories which follow, each nurse has had enough sorrows to keep her human, and enough hope to keep her happy. Even when the answers to difficult questions aren't readily available, each nurse finds a faithful friend in the medicine of life, because the questions are worth pondering.

WHO HELPS THE HELPER
- R - R - R -

Emergency room nurse Paula is one of 9,047 nurses in Saskatchewan. She draws on her considerable experience to describe some of the difficulties in dealing with grave adversity.

In the winter, two young intoxicated men in their early thirties were driving snowmobiles, and plunged through the ice into a lagoon. For a long time, the city police diving team and the firemen tried to find them, while family members anxiously waited. Many hours later both bodies were spotted and brought up to the surface.

The bodies were brought to emergency and the distraught families came in as well. When all was said and done, the men were dead and that was the end of it. It was too late for any resuscitation attempts.

But the families had to be dealt with by the nurses. They had to be comforted with compassion and cups of steaming hot coffee. They were given assistance with notifying family members and friends, calling the clergy and a funeral home. The flowers could be ordered later.

After the bodies were properly identified, the identifying toe tags had to be written out and tied with string onto the now stone-cold big toes. The bodies had to be wrapped by the nurses, dead weights rolled first to one side and then to the other, to place the white plastic shroud packs underneath and around them. And the bodies had to be lifted from the stretchers onto the morgue stretchers, covered with a sheet, and taken down in the back elevator to the morgue by the nurses. The morgue book had to be signed.

The firemen and the policemen received a debriefing session to deal with the trauma. The nurses didn't. The irony of the situation struck me. Who dealt with the families? Who wrapped the bodies in the bags? Who took them down to the morgue?

MATCHED UP
- ꓤ - ꓤ - ꓤ -

"I love every minute on the burn unit," says nurse Mary Ann in Manitoba. "And teaching kids about burns is a bonus with unbelievable rewards. I received fabulous letters from the kids — insightful and caring. The whole experience was a warm fuzzy for me."

When we took the severely burned twenty-eight-year-old patient into the burn bath, his left ear fell off and floated on top of the water solution. First, I had to make sure I didn't throw up right on the spot, and then figure out how to remove the ear without him seeing it.

I didn't want to touch it, so I grabbed a washcloth and scooped it up. Fortunately he was lying down in the bath. Our patients frequently lose bits of cartilage here and there, tips of ears or noses, but this was the whole thing. Where could I put it and what on earth was I to do with it?

His face was badly burned and the loss of his ear was one more predicament to deal with. As he progressed he, like most patients, asked to see himself in the mirror. By this time, he had already experienced looking at burns to other parts of his body, but this was troublesome.

When he woefully realized that his ear was missing, on top of the terrible burns to the rest of his face, he looked crest-fallen and said that all he had left was a hole in the side of his head. I carefully explained that while the damage to the tissues had been too great to sustain circulation to his ear, the plastic surgeons could build up an ear for him by using tissue from other parts of his body. It's a lengthy process involving numerous reconstructive procedures. This patient turned out to be lucky in this regard.

And I was lucky the week the schools had Burn Prevention Week. The teachers invited me to give a lecture on burns. I was delighted with the opportunity, but I was concerned about my slides. My own kids grew up with me working here and had their initial curiosity satisfied early on. Now it's a way of life for them. You don't have fingers? It ain't no big deal.

I talked about prevention, the different types of fires and different ways they could get burned. They already had exposure to *Stop, Drop and Roll* and fire escapes, but I talked about moving hot liquids from a stove to a table. We discussed electrical fires and hydro poles, because a couple of kids climbed the transmitters and got badly zapped. We talked about camp fires, falling asleep with a cigarette, and drinking. The majority of our burns are alcohol related.

I focused on both familiar and unfamiliar things — about people pouring gas into farm equipment, storing paint and combustible cleaners, that it's the fumes in gasoline that ignite. Then the kids had fun putting on a skit where they all pretended to be different kinds of fires.

Cosmetology is offered to our patients, so I took "before" and "after" pictures of the healing scars. I was worried the pictures would gross the kids out and discussed it with their teacher. I didn't want to scare them, but she didn't think it would be a problem.

I needn't have worried. One of the initial questions was why does it look like that? One patient had set himself on fire when he was drunk, but he didn't want to die. He had severe burns to his face, chest and arms. Even after reconstructive surgery, he had numerous contractures around his eyes, and his nose was almost nonexistent.

The kids wanted to know why his eyes were so tight, and why he only had part of his nose. Then we started talking about how he must feel. It made me a little teary-eyed to realize they were so aware and caring.

It was a wonderful experience and I have been invited back this year. I love what I do and it makes it easy to talk about.

COURAGE IS THE SUREST WISDOM
- ℞ - ℞ - ℞ -

Occasionally we encounter a nurse who is so courageous and giving, despite personal illness, that she draws others to her like a beacon in a sea of darkness.

Rose is one such Ontario nurse. She is bright, elegant, and quick. She knows she makes a difference. "I don't want anyone to feel sorry for me," she says. "That's the worst thing. Cancer patients don't want that."

After a busy shift in emergency, I was laying on the couch watching TV and I scratched my left breast — it was itchy. I felt a lump which didn't feel normal, but I thought it would go away.

Two weeks passed and it didn't go away, so I spoke to one of our surgeons and made an appointment for the following day in the clinic.

"I don't think it's anything," she said, "but let's do a needle aspiration."

After the procedure, she said she would call me if it was positive, but I was to see her in one month regardless. At that point, she said she'd feel more comfortable with a biopsy, even though the needle aspiration was negative.

She booked me right away and the biopsy and frozen section were done under general anesthetic. She was in the recovery room when I first opened my eyes. My mouth was so dry I could barely move my tongue.

"Rose," she said, "I'm sorry." I was groggy but I heard her say, "I'm sorry but it's cancer."

I fell asleep again and when I woke up I asked the nurse if I was dreaming or did the doctor really come in and tell me I had cancer. The nurse said, "I'm afraid it's true, the doctor did say you have cancer."

I couldn't believe it. I didn't know how to feel, it was such a shock. I got home before my husband. When he got there he said, "Well, you survived."

I didn't say anything. I lay down and sent both of my sons to a movie. I didn't tell them I had cancer, but I told my husband. He was dumbfounded and refused to talk about it. He kept saying, "Whoever you have to go and see, go and see. Do what you have to."

The surgeon booked my surgery for the following week. "If you can save my breast," I told her, "save it." She said some women don't want any part of their breast if they have cancer. Not me, I wanted my breast.

I had a lumpectomy and that was cancerous, but she didn't know about the nodes yet. I didn't want my husband in the recovery room waiting for me during the operation. I told him to go to work. I know what he's like.

When he came to visit me I was up already and my IV was out. The next morning I went to visit my friends in emerg. I had to stay in the hospital another two days because I had a drain inserted.

I was hoping for good news because I felt so well that day, but the surgeon said, "I think I removed all the cancer in your breast, but your pathology came back and one of the eight nodes has cancer."

Even though I'm a nurse, I didn't know much about pathology or even cancer. "What do you mean eight nodes, from where? Was one closer to the breast?"

She said, "We don't mark them, but one out of eight was positive."

"What does that mean?"

"It means your cancer wasn't localized. It has spread to the nodes, but we don't know if it went anywhere else."

She booked me for an ultrasound of the liver, a bone scan, and a liver scan to find out. She cried while we talked. The next step, she said, was to see one of the oncologists about chemotherapy and radiation.

He came in the evening. My younger son, who was only eleven years old, came to visit me with our neighbour. He was outside the door but I didn't know. I wanted to wait till I got home to tell my sons I had cancer. But while the oncologist was talking to me, my younger son was listening in the hall.

When he came in, he said, "Mummy, do you have cancer?"

"How do you know?" I asked him.

"I was outside the door when that doctor talked to you. Is that what Terry Fox had?"

Fox was dead by that time.

"Yes," I said, "but I'm going to be okay. It doesn't mean that I'm going to die like Terry Fox did."

I told him there was medicine for cancer and I'd be okay. That day was overwhelming for me, first to be told the bad news, my son's arrival, and then the oncologist telling me I needed radiation and chemotherapy.

I was worried about losing my hair — that was the biggest thing actually. The oncologist told me I'd only lose about ten percent, but I didn't believe him. Two days later I was at home, lying on the couch, and extremely depressed.

I saw another oncologist a week after my surgery. My head was reeling and I couldn't remember half or even a third of what he told me.

Consequently, I didn't know what to expect. I didn't know I would be there all day, they would do blood work, and lay me down in a little chemo room with big blue lounge chairs. They started an IV and gave me intravenous drugs.

They also gave me Ativan to relax, and told me not to drive. I agreed. After the chemo I stopped into emerg where one of my physician friends told me how terrible I looked. "Why don't you wait," he said, "and I'll drive you home."

"I'm fine," I said, and drove myself home.

I had chemotherapy treatments, one every three weeks, and each was different. My hair loss was minimal and I was the only one who was aware of it at all. The radiation started after the second chemo, every day for four weeks. That was finished in December but

Christmas was coming, and I didn't want to go back to work till after New Year's.

The biggest thing was having to drive downtown — the radiation was nothing. They put me on the table and radiated one side of the breast for two minutes. I didn't feel anything, it was like having an x-ray.

I had the purple marks for radiation. They told me not to shower or to use deodorant, but I didn't listen to them. How could I go a month without a shower? The marks washed off a bit, but they were still able to see them. I had fifty-one treatments, one every day except weekends.

Sometimes I had to go for radiation and come back for chemotherapy the same day. Radiation was finished in mid-December and chemotherapy in March.

At home, my youngest son was the only one who would talk about my treatments. He always knew when I was going for chemotherapy and asked how I was feeling. "When are you going to be finished? After the chemotherapy you won't be sick anymore, will you?"

"No, I won't," I said.

Neither my husband nor my sixteen-year-old ever mentioned chemotherapy or cancer. They ignored it and two years later they still don't talk about it. They offered to drive me, but I didn't want them to because I knew how it affected them. That was fair enough, because I had many good friends from work to talk to and to help.

I went back to work a month after my surgery, while still getting chemotherapy. I'd work a twelve hour night shift, go for my treatment, then go home to sleep.

Ironically, my first patient was a woman with breast cancer. After being diagnosed two years previously, she refused all treatment. Now she had bone metastasis and was dying.

At that time, chemotherapy was difficult for me and I asked myself why I had to go through it, when I didn't even know if it worked. The doctors do some blood work and tell you if it's okay, but they don't tell you anything about the cancer. When I saw that lady, I decided to finish my chemotherapy.

I don't know why she was my patient that first night back, but I'll never forget her. I guess it happened for the better.

The surgeon and oncologist said I did really well. One day the oncologist called and asked me to see a patient who had just had a mastectomy and wasn't coping well. "Why don't you come and talk to her?" he said.

I did. She saw that I was working and happy, even though I still had one more chemo to go, and that made her feel good.

Two weeks later my surgeon asked me to do the same for another patient. A few months later a nurse from our operating room developed cancer, had a mastectomy, and again the surgeon asked me to talk to her.

One night in emerg we had a lady with breast cancer who was on chemotherapy. She didn't know I had chemo two days before myself. She came in because of nausea and I told her I had breast cancer and how I felt. The oncologist said, "I don't think I need to be called in for a consult anymore, you're here now."

I wanted to work with oncology patients. I thought I could help. Two months after I finished chemo there was an opening for an oncology nurse in ambulatory care, but I didn't get the job. They thought I would have a hard time and didn't want to hire me. They were afraid.

I tried again. The same thing. But I was pushy and applied again. At my interview they said, "If there's a patient in a room dying of breast cancer, how would you feel?"

I said I'd feel the same as with any other patient, so they gave me a chance. I started part-time, and six months later, became full-time. Everyone saw that working in oncology and looking after patients with cancer, some of whom were dying, didn't affect me and I was able to help some of them.

I didn't tell everybody I had breast cancer. If it was going to help someone, I opened up and told them. One patient recognized me because she and I used to come for chemo at the same time.

"Look at you, doing so well," she said. "Look at me, I'm on chemotherapy again."

That made me become more selective about whom I should talk to, because I didn't want patients saying, "You're doing well and I'm dying." Since then I've only talked to patients I knew would benefit.

I prepared myself formally by getting my certificate in oncology. At one point I thought I wanted to teach. One of the oncologists said he would support me in anything I decided, but felt my work in the clinic would be missed. I've decided to remain in my present role.

I look at life differently now. For example, my oldest son wanted a car a few months after I came out of the hospital. I was in remission. I knew I wasn't cured, because there's no cure for cancer and it can come back at any time — I might die in six months. So I bought the car for him and felt good about it, but I wouldn't have if I hadn't been sick.

I take one day at a time. I know cancer can come back, but I say to myself that whatever comes, I'll deal with it. I'd like to retire when I'm fifty-five. If I'm still alive.

THE QUEST
- R - R - R -

"One hundred howling huskies sat outside my bedroom window for three days and two nights," says nurse Becky in the Yukon, "and I absolutely loved it."

During the Yukon Quest in the 1990s, the dog sledding teams ran from Alaska, down through the

Yukon, and into Whitehorse. As luck would have it, my two-nurse nursing station was situated in a gorgeous little place right on their route.

The mushers lived for the quest and never seemed to sleep. Some came into the nursing station regarding their own minor problems, but most did this as a pretext for what they really wanted. "Would you mind coming out and having a look at my dog?" they asked.

It's a good job I love dogs and am into veterinary medicine. One dog had a small laceration on his paw. Others suffered from frostbite and various minor problems.

I used my nursing skills, especially for frostbitten doggy feet. I wrapped them in flamazine dressings for the night — you can't submerge a frostbite in warm or hot water — and in the morning gently removed them.

The dogs got into scraps because they were tired, irritable and overworked. Some had travelled a few hundred miles in one day at fifty below, with the windchill factor. They were wonderful though. We had so much fun.

Naturally, I hoped the dogs I treated would win the Yukon Quest, but I loved every one of them.

Nurse, Hear You, Hear Me

A SKETCH

- R - R - R -

Mona, a nurse in the Northwest Territories, says, "It's an incredible land up here. Anyone who flies over can't believe how many hundreds of miles you can go, without seeing anything but rock and snow and water. And the people continually astound me."

Those of us who work in public health find drugs and alcohol are big problems in the north. Addiction programs and rehab centres are available, and we have a program for teens to deal with solvent abuse. Tuberculosis, sexually transmitted diseases, and nutrition are other major areas of concern.

We have a literacy program and every new baby gets a T-shirt with eight languages printed on the back, as well as little books. We encourage parents to read to their children.

Our prenatal classes are huge. We run them all the time because it's a young population here and the doctors promote our classes. Right now we have classes running four nights a week, after our day shift, so it's hectic.

We're trying to have more birthing in the nursing stations because it can be lonely for mothers who have to leave home. They used to have birthing in the stations when British and Australian midwives worked here.

The nurses up in the high Arctic are isolated in the nursing stations. They can be weathered in for days. Fortunately the planes are faster now and communication is better. Most settlements have nice airports, unlike the strips of gravel when I first came here.

The people are wonderful and appreciative. The nurses deserve praise because they work hard and are on call twenty-four hours a day. Still, anyone who has worked in the north would never want to go down south, where a doctor has to give permission to give an aspirin.

RECIPE FOR FAILURE
- ℞ - ℞ - ℞ -

"When I graduated as a clinical nurse specialist in Ontario," says Irene, "I was energized in caring for people who were cognitively impaired, and was particularly interested in the phenomenon of agitation with cognitively impaired elders. This is a story of successes and failures."

I had to establish my credibility with staff who were much more experienced in all of this than I was. I introduced myself.

"Are there any particular patients you're feeling challenged by and would like me to help with?" I asked.

The first comment was, "If she can do something with Joseph Galston, we'll really be happy." I thought this must be a recipe for failure.

I found him to be profoundly agitated. He was sitting in a wheelchair, ineffectively rolling it with a back and forth movement on his wheels and sometimes shuffling his feet. "JAMES ... JAMES ... JAMES," he called out continually.

When he was quiet, he still rolled his wheels back and forth in the hallway, in fairly public view.

The other problem was his hostility and combativeness toward nurses giving his morning care. He swore and swung his arms at them and they were afraid of coming to harm. I felt particularly challenged.

When I started working with him it wasn't at an intellectual level. I began at a physical response level, bringing some lotion with me. I was really experimenting with this person in terms of my own nursing research, because I wasn't going to recommend something to the staff if it wasn't going to work. And I didn't know what was going to work, because there was nothing systematic in the literature.

I sat down in a wheelchair beside him and did some work with my body to indicate a measured pacing with him, monitoring my movements with him, in some sort of rhythm.

"What I'd like to do is to help you relax," I said, and put some lotion on his arm so that it was not abrasive to him.

He started to calm down. Whether I was deliberately pacing him down or not I'm not sure — that's my intellectual analysis coming out — but he did calm down.

That seemed to be a breakthrough in a way — we were able to establish a rapport. I went through the social amenities afterward, introducing myself. I didn't load him with verbiage at this initial reception.

I was aware of the fact that I would want to be treated in a specific way, if it were me. I came in to do his care on several consecutive days. The curtains in the room were drawn. "Good morning, Mr. Galston," I said, "it's Brenda Duneau. I'm going to open the curtains now."

I did that slowly because there are two ways to open curtains — quick and startling, or slow and relaxing.

For each step of his care I told him what I was going to do before I did it. We sailed through our first encounter. Priscilla, his primary nurse, who was sure I would fail, wondered what I had done.

I didn't do anything remarkable — I engaged in social amenities. I didn't do anything more powerful than that.

In going through his chart what was astounding to me was the number of losses this man had had in a short period of time. In two years, this eighty-year-old man had moved three or four times. When his wife became disabled, they moved so she could be accommodated, and she died shortly thereafter.

He fractured his hip and could no longer cope. Another move and another hospitalization followed. Then his nephew suggested he move closer to him — all within two years. He was functional and had been making family decisions, but now his behaviours had decompensated.

This is a man who had been vice-president of a large corporation, had held a responsible position, and engaged internationally with incredible social grace. His repertoire of skills was profound.

An exquisitely beautiful picture on his bedside table provided the clues. It was a wonderful photograph, probably taken in the early 1900s, showing his wife as a bride. There was wealth, privilege, intellect, and the unimaginable reserve this man had come with, and expectations to social engagement.

For me, the whole notion of personhood became pre-eminent. How would we engross this man now?

If there was a way of devaluing a person who had probably been addressed as "Mister" most of his life, to call him "Joe" would certainly do that, and some staff members did.

I was passionate in wanting to bring forth the best in this man. I didn't think anything of substance had happened in terms of his intellect, but once anyone has been labelled as demented, that's a powerful label to overcome.

I told Priscilla what I was doing, hoping she might try the same thing. She did, before going on vacation for two weeks. A significant amount of time.

When she returned Mr. Galston said, "Where have you been?"

"He does know what's going on here," she told me.

After that we were able to demonstrate to the staff that he was capable of much more appropriate behaviour, but he needed to be approached in a way that recognized his intellect.

We got him to the point where he was continent of stool because his needs were being listened to, but we were not able to have him continent of urine. Then he was transferred to a different floor with different staff.

If I had realized, I would have altered my approach. Here I was, a novice clinical nurse specialist (CNS), being respectful of the institution and its boundaries. I laid the groundwork the best I could with the staff and the CNS on his new floor to make a good transition for him. But within a week of being there, he fell. Once again he was labelled as aggressive.

I didn't know how to deal with this predicament. For some reason, I could not get through to the other CNS about the abilities this man had demonstrated. I think it was my inexperience, but I felt powerless. At that point, I moved to another city and for me, this was crashing down.

I know now I would have conditions for a person to be considered a successful transfer to another unit. I'd work with the new staff, and the patient, as opposed to handing him over. I can't sink to recrimination or place any blame on the accepting staff, and so I bear the burden.

HEART OF GOLD
- ℞ - ℞ - ℞ -

Lisette, an operating room nurse in Quebec, specializes in heart transplants, and explains the process from the nurse's point of view.

When we first started, we didn't know how families would react to their relatives having a heart that belonged to somebody else. They were at the OR door all the time asking questions.

Many nurses weren't comfortable with the idea of doing heart transplants, but after gaining experience, this changed. Now it's easier for all of us to deal with.

We understand the purpose of the surgery and we are dealing with our own emotions. Some of the nurses had prejudices because they didn't think it was the right thing to do on some occasions — sometimes they were transplanting a sixty-year-old heart into a forty-year-old patient, and the typical questions that arose were disconcerting and problematic.

With classes and in-service, the more difficult aspects have eased somewhat. One problem was how to deal with the donor's body after the procedure, because there's nothing left. Nurses were in a quandary trying to cope.

If we needed to talk following surgery, some of the alternatives we were given were pastoral care, taking a break, and talking amongst ourselves. We asked the surgeons to be respectful, because once the surgery is done, they leave everything and the nurse has to extubate the patient and complete the rest of the care.

Most of the time the donors are from this hospital, making it easier because we don't have to wait. They sometimes come from another hospital, and that is notably stressful for us.

We started heart surgery more than ten years ago. We had done some previous to that, but they were not successful. There are now no OR nurses here who have not been able to come to terms with doing heart transplants.

It was tough when we started having patients with AIDS, because as nurses, some of us didn't want to have anything to do with them, because we were afraid ourselves. We didn't know how to protect ourselves, or what to do, but we are all continually learning. We don't know if a patient has AIDS. We work with universal precautions and everyone is treated the same.

What is sometimes troublesome for nurses has been the restraint in costs. It's difficult to work with limited resources and try to be innovative at the same time. We have to teach ourselves and we have to teach the surgeons to be aware, because they don't know how much things cost. Here we are the centre for transplants. That's expensive, so we have to cut costs somewhere else.

We can do a heart transplant with two nurses. Besides the anesthetist, there are two doctors and usually a student because we're a teaching hospital. This is straightforward. A heart transplant is easier to do than a coronary bypass because there's less suturing, just four vessels.

Liver transplants take five or six hours, but some require up to twenty hours if they bleed or have other problems. Obviously more nurses are needed then. On average, we do one liver transplant per month, but just before Christmas, we did five.

Here in the province of Quebec we have a transplant bank which organizes transplants so they know which patient has priority. If it's our turn, then we get them. If not, then it's for another hospital.

MINISTRY OF TALENTS
- R - R - R -

Ruthanne is a nurse who changed professions and is now a minister of the United Church in Ontario.

"I've always thought of my journey from nursing into the ministry as being a little bit like a tapestry. One piece got picked up and then another and another, so it's hard to know where the origin was," she explains.

When I first graduated I worked in an outpost in northern Manitoba. There were no roads, so we flew up there. There was a real sense of community. The amount of responsibility I had was scary. I went from being a little dot in the whole system, to being one of the major components. I became aware of the phenomenal poverty level that exists in Canada for the native people.

I left the north with the intent of returning after getting additional training in ICU. Once there, however, my journey into the ministry began with a series of questions.

I had many critical patients and it came to me that I didn't know what my personal theology about life was. I was dealing with issues I wasn't sure about in my own mind, and needed to know more about.

My own father developed cancer of the pancreas and I returned to Ontario to care for him. I tried to help my mother cope with the reality that he wasn't going to get better, and questioned the idea of trying treatments in Mexico. Where do we start and end the process, the sense of promoting life, or giving it up to death?

When he died several months later I went through the usual textbook stages of grief and felt a lot of anger. The same questions arose — what did I believe about life and death?

I went back out west as a VON nurse. I liked the individual care I could give and met one particularly interesting woman. She had suffered through many hardships during her life and had severe arthritis. What struck me wasn't her illness, but her hope and her strength. There are some people who can take on tremendous loads of responsibility and maintain a spirit of health and hope. She was one of them.

I realized there was a real mystery about life and death, and about pain and illness. I believe there's a lot more to life and living than the day-to-day things.

In nursing, we get the whole gamut of life right in front of us on any given day. We experience someone dying, being born, and dealing with acute illness. The mystery of beginnings and endings has always puzzled me. These elements made me realize I needed to know more, to get my questions answered.

I obtained my B.A. in Religious Studies, and took a course in chaplaincy, where ministers are trained in institution ministry. I wasn't ordained yet, but they allowed me to come in because of my nursing experience.

For one year I was responsible for the spiritual well-being of patients on a psycho-geriatric ward, most of whom had alzheimers. Consequently I was dealing more with staff and family.

A whole door opened to me and people told me how they felt about their lives, their spirit, and God. They asked me for information that wasn't accessible from being a nurse. I realized then that I wanted to care for people's souls.

My nursing experience has been invaluable in my ministry, especially in being able to relate to people, and to have a sense of ease in various environments. I still do a quick head-to-toe assessment, but now for a different reason.

Hospital equipment doesn't threaten me and I can be more comfortable for the other person. People in my congregation have said their connecting point with me is my nursing. Either they are nurses or somebody in their family is. In the midst of all this I had cancer myself and went for chemotherapy. People realize I know something about living in fear.

I was asked to do some work on a congregation that wasn't well. A congregation can be sick in the same way a human being can. There may be friction between the ministers, and the resulting breakdown is the same as having our immune system break down. It clicked in that an assessment, diagnosis, and treatment were required, so nursing skills are definitely transferable to the ministry.

On a bad day, I wonder why I ever left nursing, but I know nursing is not easy these days. If nurses just had to worry about the care of individual patients, that would be okay, but the institutional stresses are excessive.

THE PRESENT MOMENT
- ℞ - ℞ - ℞ -

"I'm a nephrology specialist," says Alberta nurse Eileen. "I try to instill hope in people because a positive attitude goes a long way. Intuition also plays a large part in my care."

A young boy celebrated his sixteenth birthday with a cocktail of antifreeze given to him by his friends. He went into kidney failure and had to be dialyzed on what was probably the first dialysis machine in Canada. It was like a great big washing machine. This unconscious kid was semi-naked, with tubes everywhere. I was in absolute awe of the procedure. He died.

Later, I had a twenty-one-year-old patient dying of kidney failure — Bright's Disease, or glomerulonephritis. Uremic frost glistened on his face. All we could do was restrict his fluids and wait. When he died, I covered him up with a sheet.

The dialysis unit was ten months old by this time and everyone was terrified of it. I decided to take the six-week training period required to work there, with the proviso that if I didn't like it, I could leave.

The tank and keel kidney I started working with was massive. I would run four patients by myself, two of them deathly ill. There were times I crawled under the bed because I couldn't get past the patients with all their lines.

One night I had a patient hooked up to the dialysis machine with blood running through the keel, or dialyzer, when the machine started smoking. I unplugged it and took the patient off dialysis. Fires were common and our approach was common sense.

Changes in technology meant learning and adapting. Community machines replaced the single ones. We had to measure all the chemicals, pour them into the tank, fill it with water, and mix it. The pipes from the tank connected to every person who was in dialysis. Sometimes the pipes broke and the mixture poured over everybody's head. One nurse dropped a beaker into the tank, crawled in to clean it up, and couldn't get out.

As I looked at all the people who were attached to machines because their lives depended on it, many questions went through my mind — if you've got ten years, is this the way you want to live? What kind of a life are you going to have? Are you going to see your children grow up? Are you going to know the love of another person? What is your experience in life going to be?

Although these people had limitations, I felt I could help them transcend their illnesses, to capture some of the beauty in their lives, and to depart with more precious experiences.

I put a lot of energy and time and effort to help people come to grips with the fact that, yes, their kidneys weren't working. No, they didn't feel energetic. Yes, they often felt sick. But what about the cherished moments? Would they rather be dead? Or would they rather be alive?

Instilling a sense of independence in my patients was always important to me. Initially only doctors were allowed to needle the areas of artificial tubing underneath the patients' skin to attach them to a machine. Then they taught me.

When I saw how easy it was I decided to teach these skills to our patients. We got the seal of approval and in the next month we sent five patients home on dialysis. After that, they never let us touch them. They became independent and took a lot of pride in what they did for themselves. I loved the challenge of teaching the ones who were unteachable, because they always ended up with a feeling of control over their lives.

Before we had enough knowledge to know what immunosuppression would do and at what level it could cause major problems, we used a lot of heavy artillery. Many young people in their twenties died from volatile disease caused by immunosuppression. That tore my soul apart. Right now, we have a ninety percent success rate.

Patients waiting for kidney transplants hope their lives will change, and they do, dramatically. I rejoice with them when they're restored to health. The joy is incredible.

One of my patients was dialyzed three times a week, five hours each time, for nineteen years, and maintained a full-time job. When an opportunity for a transplant came, he was hopeful that things would work out, but terrified that they might not. His reaction was typical of all transplant patients.

When transplants don't work out, and ten percent of them don't, I go through the pain and sorrow of each experience because it's like another death. It's the death of the organ and the death of hope. This can happen immediately, or after someone has had the transplant for years. Then they have to go back on dialysis.

The patients go through the grieving process and try to understand it — denial, anger, bargaining, grieving, and acceptance. But grieving is grieving, regardless of the cause.

I have known some of these patients for years. When they're hurting, I'm hurting. I've seen their tears. I've wept with them. I've hugged them. I've been part of their weddings. I've been part of their children growing up. I've been part of their life experience.

One patient was a married man in his thirties. He had a type of disease in which the possibility of recurrence into a transplanted kidney existed. While the chances were slight, it could happen with great rapidity.

We let him know all the risks. The decision was to go ahead with a transplant from a family member. We transplanted the kidney and within twenty-four hours, there was a volatile recurrence of his original disease.

Feeling the family's pain was heartbreaking. We had to put forth a plan to them, not knowing what the outcome would be — not even really knowing what the plan was. But things turned around. His kidney function returned, and with it, hope returned.

Some doctors laugh when I say this, but people who come with a positive attitude and feel that things are going to work out okay often see the realization of their hopes. Others come with a sense that something just isn't together, and many times it isn't. I think attitude does play a part.

As a nurse, I try to enhance the quality of life. I use every technique possible, whatever works, including visualization. "What can you see yourself doing in fifteen years time?" I ask.

"I'm not going to be alive."

And I say, "And what if you are? What are you going to do with your life? What are you going to do in five years? What do you want to do by the end of this year? You can't plan for tomorrow, but you can dream about tomorrow, and you can live for today."

My patients have given me so much. The biggest learning experience is how to live one day at a time. I plan for the future, but I live right now. I look at the trees right now. I hug my cats right now. I enjoy my parents right now. I live right in the moment.

ENTREPRENEUR
— R — R — R —

Like Ed Mirvish, who founded the world's first discount department store, nurse Tammy is filling a need.
"In the last ten months," she explains, "I've been working on starting my own business, a retirement home service for seniors here in Ontario."

I have my first customers and that's tremendously exciting. As administrator of a seniors' home for the last three years, I saw how many seniors did not want to leave their homes. They came in kicking and screaming, even at ninety. Their sons or daughters insisted, even though the seniors were very reluctant. I decided to offer the same services as the seniors' home, but in the person's own home.

I have a good roster of competent and reliable people that I know and trust to provide the necessary services. I'm careful of who I send in, because it has to be a good match. My computer will soon match the services required with the person available to provide that service.

The services range from homemaking to snow shovelling, to making meals, food shopping, dry cleaning, hairdressing, a live-in homemaker, you name it. Anything they want, I can provide. If their fridge breaks down, I can arrange to have it repaired, just like I would in a retirement home.

There's only one payment per month, and I'm responsible for everything. The seniors know exactly what they're paying for, and can plan their finances. They often worry about writing cheques and many don't see all that well.

I keep in touch with my clients to make sure they're all right. Even on days we don't go in, I phone them to see how they're doing. I love this aspect of the business.

Advertising is by word-of-mouth because I don't want to overspend. Ninety percent of businesses go under in the first year because of overhead, so I'm being careful.

I'd like to get a few good customers, do everything properly, and then grow. I'm giving myself a year to inject quality into the business before advertising on a large scale.

I've targeted an affluent area in the city where many seniors are concentrated. If this works, franchising may be an interesting option. Every little step forward is exciting.

HAIR TODAY
- ℞ - ℞ - ℞ -

Nurse Therese works and lives among the Inuit in the far reaches of Quebec. "I've been working here long enough to accept things that others would consider unusual," she says. "This is my adopted culture."

Women here who are sick and can't quite pinpoint their problem have a unique treatment. They cut their hair very short, and then as it grows back, they believe that their strength grows back at the same time. Even women with beautiful long hair will cut it, but stop short of completely shaving it right off. It frequently works for them, rather like pruning a plant.

Someone in the family usually does the honours, but some do cut their own hair. Younger women who live with their mothers or grandmothers always keep this habit, even if I give them antibiotics or other medication. I have never tried this for myself, but many of my Inuit friends swear by it.

Lillian R. Tymchuk, RN

VALUES AND LIFESTYLES
- ℞ - ℞ - ℞ -

"AIDS has profoundly impacted on nurses here," reflects Elaine in Ontario. *"Apart from the gay staff, most of us have never examined various values and lifestyles, whatever our inclinations or prejudices. We hit this head-on, so it had to change us."*

I've worked in palliative care for some time, caring primarily for gay men who have AIDS. Their psychosocial problems are devastating and there's always trauma.

We see partners. Because our place is small, we deal with people who accompany the patients far more than would be the case in any hospital.

When Roger, Jack's partner of fourteen years, brought him in, he couldn't take care of him at home any longer. Every day Roger came here from work in his business suit. He'd take his jacket off, roll up his sleeves, and take total care of Jack until 11:00 P.M. Jack was incontinent, vomiting, and difficult to care for. Some days he knew Roger, some days he didn't. Although exhausted, Roger never wavered. He altered my perceptions.

George's brothers and sisters came from a strong religious persuasion. In his late forties, George had a neurological disorder causing him to have outbursts of vile language plus a nasty temper, much like Turret's syndrome.

When his family came in he would be spouting this offensive language. Imagine their pain as they tried to find a way to reach him, to come to terms with their own feelings, and to decide what they should and shouldn't do.

We had to do a good deal of intervention for the family not to take George's behaviour personally and we worked at explaining the disease process. We told them that although George's primary nurse had been close to him, George turned on her too, but he didn't know what he was doing. In the end they did resolve their feelings. We were happy to see him hang on long enough for that to happen.

We do have counsellors, but they're almost never here in the evenings, and that's when most families come in. So counselling is part of our job too. Many of our staff, myself included, come from a background in psychiatric nursing and have taken additional courses. We've all had life experiences involving loss.

Working here changes the way we as nurses look at the meaning of life. We re-examine our own values, what's important in life, and how we treat others. Our tolerance levels are altered as we change and grow.

Ninety percent of our patients are admitted with dementia, and Charlie, a man in his early forties, was no exception. He wasn't aware of his condition so he wasn't unhappy on that account.

He had three close male friends, at least one of whom came in every single day for a month. They took total care of him, changing him, feeding him, and giving him whirlpool baths. They brought wine and had nice meals with him. They became close to us.

Then one of the three men was brutally murdered. I didn't realize it initially because he went by his middle name, and the media used his first name. The paper said he had been known to frequent homosexual bars. He had been dead for two days before being found.

We were devastated. The media helps form people's attitudes, and the implication was that this wasn't an important murder, that he probably had it coming. There's no need for an attitude that allows the rest of us to dismiss him. We lit a candle for him.

FOUR

HUMOUR - NO LAUGHING MATTER
- ℞ - ℞ - ℞ -

A merry heart doeth good like a medicine.

Proverbs 17:22

Nurses use laughter and humour to deflate the harsher realities of life and periodically to take a back-handed swipe at Death. Many terrible shifts have been turned into satisfying ones for both the patient and nurse through the use of humour. A merry heart literally opens up the body's ability to cope with the burdensome stresses which serious illness and ordinary living impose, in real and physically measurable ways.

Laughter, when it opens up an entire upper level on which to relate and to communicate and to heal, is a spiritual gift which must be accepted and shared with thanksgiving. Laughter is contagious, and like music, a delight that is bestowed effortlessly and without the encumbrances of language.

Writer Norman Cousins claims that laughter is a form of internal jogging that enhances respiration, moves internal organs around, and is an igniter of great expectations. The latter aspect is the most important, for only with great expectations can great things come.

Time is a celebrated ally which allows the amusement buried deep in most situations to make itself known. Great comedy is said to be tragedy plus time. Part of the real joy of laughter, which may be anything from a tiny titter to a resounding roar, lies in the shared remembrance of a funny story. Laughter is never lonely.

The incidents that follow are ones in which Canadian nurses found something to laugh at. Often they laughed at themselves.

PRACTICAL JOKER
- ℞ - ℞ - ℞ -

"I was noted for playing practical jokes" says Curtis, one of 208 nurses in the Yukon. "But some people don't consider what happened one night a joke, even though they still tell the story at Christmas parties. They think I should have been fired."

It was the dead of winter after six months in the Yukon. My evening shift on the medical ward was quietly winding up.

I decided to make up a fictitious mental health admission and encouraged the two CNAs on my shift to go along with me. We didn't have a separate psychiatric ward, but on my floor we had Room Four, which was a locked room.

Every hospital has a Resusci-Annie, a dummy on which to practice CPR, and she became my patient in Room Four. I dimmed the lights and partially covered her with a blanket.

All the mental health forms, including a Commissioners' Form complete with his signature, chart, and medication cards, were neatly organized for the night shift.

With a straight face I gave report at midnight. I said we had a thirty-five-year-old woman who tried to kill her husband with an axe. She was in Room Four but under no circumstances were they to go in there without an RCMP escort — this was the usual protocol. In the morning she was to be transferred to Vancouver with an RCMP escort.

The new grad's eyes widened with anticipation of a troublesome shift. My expectation was that in half an hour, after first rounds, the joke would be over. I went home to bed and forgot about it, not even bothering to tell my wife.

However, as I later learned, when the night staff made their first rounds they peeked into Room Four and saw a sleeping patient with her face toward the wall. They watched intently to make sure she was breathing and decided she must be okay.

When the supervisor came by she was quite concerned she hadn't been told anything about this patient on her report. She was responsible for making arrangements for the morning transfer and decided to call the admitting doctor for additional information — the name of one of our regular doctors was on the chart. His response was, "I don't have time for this," and he hung up on her.

In the meantime, the night nurses had done rounds again, and reported that this patient had turned over and was sleeping on her opposite side.

By now the supervisor was getting in a major snit. She called the RCMP and told them to come to the hospital. The corporal on duty, who happened to be a friend of mine, didn't know anything about it and he hung up on her too. She called the RCMP inspector and complained about the uncooperativeness of the local RCMP.

The inspector called the corporal and had him wake up all the officers who had worked the evening shift to find out who had brought this patient in. Many of these were my friends and neighbours.

Numerous phone calls later, the corporal phoned the supervisor back and said, "Look, NOBODY knows anything about your patient in Room Four."

At four o'clock in the morning I got a phone call. My explanation resulted in absolute silence on the other end of the phone, prior to a loud CLICK! I went upstairs and told my wife, who also is an RN, that we probably would be leaving the Yukon shortly.

The next evening I fully expected to be brought up on the carpet by the director of nursing, but nobody said boo. The reason was that the nurses had charted that the patient was breathing, had rolled over, and had good colour.

It was a good six months before the supervisor even spoke to me, and certain other people refused to recognize the humour. I decided never again to play any practical jokes.

As time wore on, however, I felt there could be no harm in saying I had a patient bleeding profusely from his stomach, and maybe putting a few rotten, black bananas around to look like old blood. In half an hour the joke would be over, wouldn't it?

THE MOTEL
- R - R - R -

Newfoundland nurse Pamela, who is also a midwife, discovered she had developed quite a reputation on the east coast after a certain delivery.

In Newfoundland, a well organized system to do medi-vacs was already in place when I arrived as staff nurse in obstetrics. We were ready to go anytime.

We received a call from a hospital in Quebec. They were sending a lady with her sixteenth pregnancy for a Caesarean section to avoid possible complications. They couldn't fly her over because the weather was out, so she was coming by ship. She was to be accompanied by a nurse named Shirley, but they wanted a midwife to meet her here.

It was my day off so I was dispatched with this driver to travel the thirty miles to where the ship would dock. We used stationwagons rather than ambulances. They were rattletraps, but at least we could put a stretcher in the back.

The ship had docked by the time we arrived. Shirley reported that the patient, an enormous lady by the name of Nadine, had travelled well and thankfully was not in labour. The idea of a pleasant return journey satisfied me.

Shirley and I scrunched in next to the driver. Nadine was on a stretcher in the back where I had heaped most of my equipment. The green oxygen cylinder, I decided, would be safer in an upright position between my feet.

This was September and the roads were muddy with permanently embedded tire marks underneath. As we chatted back and forth Nadine was giving little groans and moans. I thought she would soon go into labour, something I had a sense of, nothing specific — but Shirley disagreed.

"Step on it," I said to the driver, "or you'll have four passengers instead of three."

As the words came out of my mouth the stationwagon sputtered, spun in an outright revolution, and plunged down a ten-foot embankment, nose first. My glasses flew off, hit the windshield, and disappeared from view.

122

After what seemed like eons the vehicle shuddered and stopped. All was silent save a slight hissing noise. We were stunned.

The hissing persisted. I felt a cool draft on my leg and realized the oxygen cylinder was leaking. I pushed open the door, plunked the cylinder upright in the mud, and hastily turned the dial to OFF.

The stationwagon was slanted in such a way that the two wheels on the right stuck wildly in the air. Nadine had slipped off the stretcher and was lying on her left side, moaning. I proceeded round the vehicle and crawled in through a broken rear window — being tiny has its advantages.

A cursory examination showed a swollen contusion on Nadine's face and several scratches on her left arm. Otherwise she seemed all right, no obvious injuries to her abdomen. My glasses stared at me from under the stretcher.

Shirley and I hadn't really assessed our injuries or the driver's to any extent, but that was a low priority at this point. Nadine was the one who required a complete examination. I found my obstetrical bag and examined her. She was almost fully dilated, ready to have her sixteenth baby. She could sneeze and deliver, barring complications. I had no desire for a high-risk delivery in the back of an upended stationwagon, stuck in a ditch.

There wasn't much traffic on this stranded road stuck way out in the boonies, but Shirley and the driver climbed up the embankment to look for traffic. There was none.

Shirley was vaguely familiar with this area. "I think there's a motel close by," she yelled down to me, "but I'm not sure."

The sound of sputtering and a low rumble caught our attention. From my vantage point I could see a worn down, rusty old truck making its way toward us. Shirley waved frantically and the truck creaked to a stop. Two ancient men indicated they would help us. I thought I heard them say the motel was three miles away, but it was actually thirteen.

We lifted the moaning Nadine back onto the stretcher and up the embankment. The truck had oil drums in the back but there was no time to roll them off. "Put her on top of the drums," I commanded.

To this day I do not know how we did it, because she weighed at least two hundred and fifty awkward, pregnant pounds. "Please don't push," I pleaded. Beads of perspiration were pooling on her forehead.

Nadine was incredible. She did her level best not to push, while I held her hand and prayed silently, perched precariously as we were on top of the oil drums. Each passing bump inspired a new devotion.

Around a lengthy curve, in the middle of a clearing, a workers' camp came into view. We stopped and the driver phoned the hospital asking for a doctor to meet us at the motel. I was concerned about the baby because Nadine was Rhesus positive with antibodies.

After a few more miles we pulled into a small driveway in front of the motel, amidst the clanging and banging of the rolling oil drums.

Shirley ran ahead demanding a room. "We're having a baby. Give us a room. Quick." The astonished lady at the desk motioned for us to come in.

With the help of the ancient men, we carried a now panting Nadine into the tiniest room imaginable. As soon as we plunked the stretcher down on the bed I started an IV. The possibility of hemorrhage was all too real.

The obstetrics bag had so much equipment that anyone could have done a Caesarian section. Now, however, I could not find a pair of scissors or forceps to deliver this baby with. At that exasperating moment an obstetrician walked in.

"GO AND WASH YOUR HANDS," Shirley yelled.

The poor doctor was so startled that he did as he was told. In the meantime I found the necessary equipment to deliver the arriving baby and handed him over to Shirley.

The doctor returned and helped with the infant. I delivered the placenta, and we got all tidied up. The time had come to proceed to our original destination.

The doctor had driven an ambulance to the motel. First the stationwagon, then the truck with the rolling oil drums, and now this ambulance — with the red cross on the side, it looked exactly like a jeep from "MASH." I nearly collapsed with laughter.

WET AND GOOEY
- ℞ - ℞ - ℞ -

Anne loves nursing on pediatrics in Manitoba and has been known to play a joke or two on her small charges. She enjoys herself equally when she's on the receiving end.

On the peds surgery floor, in the front of each of the rooms, are plastic slots on the wall for the binders which contain patient charts. The charts slide in from the top.

One night I was making rounds at three in the morning and had to check the temperature of one particular child again. Both kids in that room were nine years old. They weren't with us too long before they started to move around and get into trouble. On my last rounds, however, they were sleeping like angels.

I reached into the slot to get the chart and felt something wet and gooey. Pushing my hand in a bit farther I met with more of the yukko stuff. Definitely time for my trusty flashlight.

The high beam showed the chart holder was three-quarters full of green Jello that slipped and slopped all over the floor as I scrambled to pick it up. It must have taken me a good hour to get rid of the melting mess since the plastic holder was screwed to the wall and I couldn't pour the Jello out.

After a few minutes of cleaning up this mess, I worried that my giggling would wake the kids up. I went in to check the temperature of the one boy, and found both of them snickering under their covers. They weren't sleeping after all.

"Now, I don't want to find another mess on the floor when I come in tonight, boys," I said.

"Okay, nurse," they promised.

The next night the boys kept exchanging glances and laughing every time they saw me.

"No mess on the floor tonight, boys. Remember. You promised."

It wasn't until my 6:00 A.M. rounds that I discovered the source of their merriment. The boys had kept their promise. There was no mess on the floor. Stuck to the ceiling with peanut butter were seven dark brown Oreo cookies.

WHY HAVE SEX?
- R - R - R -

When two sisters are both nurses in Ontario, like Wendy and Tina are, you can bet they share humourous experiences.

This is what happened to my sister, Tina, who is a public health nurse like I am. She was giving a talk in a classroom on sex to quite a young age group, grades four and five.

Mrs. Carpenter was the homeroom teacher, a pleasant, older lady. Mrs. Carpenter was standing at the back of the classroom, no doubt overjoyed that someone else was taking over her class for even a brief period.

Tina got through all the questions from the children. Then one little kid put up his hand and asked, "But WHY do people have sex?"

Startled by the question, Tina looked around for help. Who should she see but the inattentive Mrs. Carpenter looking out the window.

"Mrs. Carpenter, why do people have sex?"

All eyes were on her. Like she's the great expert on why people have sex.

"Pardon me?"

"Why do people have sex?"

She came up with a beautiful, appropriate answer that Tina said she couldn't have thought of at the time, about two people loving each other and wanting to feel as close as possible.

"Thank you, Mrs. Carpenter."

WHAT'S IN A NAME
- R - R - R -

Quebec nurse Danielle thought that orientating Claude, the new grad, to the operating room that morning was going to be routine, but was she in for a surprise.

Claude was a brand new operating room nurse who was starting his orientation. He scrubbed in on a vascular case.

128

When the surgeon was ready for the Gerald forceps, he said, "Can I have the Gerald please?"

Claude didn't respond.

"Can I have the Gerald?"

No response.

After the third time, the surgeon snapped, "GERALD PLEASE."

Claude said, "My name is Claude, not Gerald."

Claude didn't know what the forceps were. All of us, including the surgeon, had tears streaming down our faces from laughing with our colleague.

SO YOU THINK CANCER IS SERIOUS
- R̶ - R̶ - R̶ -

Alberta nurse Janet has always been known as "the funny nurse" wherever she has worked. "I've used humour myself to cope with various stresses," she says, "so naturally it's a tool I use with others."

I work on an oncology floor, which isn't a place where anyone expects much humour. However, I find that most people are already using humour as a coping skill. I read my patients' cues to see if they use humour in certain anxiety- provoking situations, or to respond to me as a nurse. If they do, then I take the lead, usually during admission or nursing procedures.

Constipation is a common occurrence on our floor because of all the narcotics given for pain control.

One man was really frustrated because he wasn't able to poop. We did the regular laxative routine, gave him a fleet enema, and then a soap suds enema. Nothing worked. "What you need is a garden hose," I joked.

In one of the housekeeping rooms was a garden hose type of attachment. I rigged it up to an IV pole, filled a large bucket with water, and walked into his room.

"Okay," I said nonchalantly. "Turn over on your side and let's get this going."

His eyes nearly popped out of his head, obviously taking me seriously. When he realized what was going on he roared with laughter until tears streamed down his face. Each time any family member or visitor came in he repeated the story with renewed gusto. He was still constipated, but at least he was able to laugh about it.

Pain control and nausea are two of our biggest problems. Sometimes it doesn't seem to matter what we do, nothing helps. It's distressing for patients and their significant others that we aren't able to do anything.

One lady had intractable vomiting and didn't respond to anything we gave her. She continued to vomit into the basin every hour on the hour. I was getting frustrated and decided to troubleshoot with one of my colleagues.

We knew that naming pain makes it concrete and easier to deal with. We simply transferred this concept to the problem of her vomiting, and decided what better item to name than her K-basin.

"You're spending so much time with your K-basin," I said to her, "why don't you give it a name?"

Ralph it was.

When her visitors came in, she'd say, "Have you met my new friend Ralph?" and she'd present the K-basin. Being able to joke about her vomiting took the pressure off an uncomfortable situation, from both herself and her visitors.

People are always relieved when a person is able to share some humour with them because they share a firm bond. A lot of significant others don't feel it's appropriate to use humour — they need a guide to realize it's okay. Humour never cures anything, but it eases many situations.

There are no limits to what I'll do to make my patients laugh — put an arrow through my head or wear a chicken suit. I admit to taking pot shots at myself, but I never ridicule others.

Humour helps people rise above their circumstances. Research shows that physically, humour and laughter are beneficial and are being used in pain control. There are multiple benefits both psychologically and physiologically.

Because I have always been known as "the funny one," I can get away with quite a bit. Once I dressed up as a witch for Halloween and was in charge at the desk. I ended up having to start an IV at a patient's bedside in this getup.

I usually let patients lead the way. Being fairly intuitive, I can figure out someone else's sense of humour. One lady, newly diagnosed with leukemia, was getting a diuretic, and as a result, had to go to the bathroom.

When I put her on the commode she overfilled it and urine went all over the floor. She was extremely embarrassed. I came in with a huge bucket and told her she could use it the next time. She laughed so hard her anxiety disappeared.

I'm currently completing a humour room and I've designed a humour cart that's taken around the unit by our volunteer clown. The cart has various hand-held toys, yo-yo's, little puzzles and bubble-blowers, all easily manipulated items. We have funny books and videos. I find that both teenagers and adults like to play.

Our hospital has a humour channel. It's on a patients' network so they can access it whether or not they buy the TV service. Funny programs are shown twice a day for two hours. TV doesn't appeal to everyone, but I know people really love the humour cart.

These incentives brought out the humour in nurses I work with, including those who were having difficulty incorporating humour with professionalism. I've done a lot of teaching about humour in our facility and it helps prevent burnout. The work load seems lighter when we're laughing and we feel better.

We have patients in the terminal stages of cancer and it's wonderful for them to hear the sound of laughter. The daughter of one told me how pleasing it was to come out of her father's room and hear someone having a good time.

For some, there is a stigma to the idea of illness and laughter, and especially to cancer and laughter. At least eighty percent of the patients I look after use humour to survive.

One young man told me he thought I was acting like a twelve-year-old because I was wearing a chicken hat. But as the day wore on he came to respect me because I dared to wear something like that. He had a tumour on his leg and although it was difficult, he decided to walk to the bathroom.

"I'll get you a urinal," I offered.

"I don't need a urinal."

I lined up ten urinals against the window and said, "This might inspire you. You can do target practice. The extra challenge might make you feel more comfortable."

Humour helps, even on a "weekend from Hell" when we don't have time to give the quality of care we want to.

BALL ROOM
- ♫ - ♫ - ♫ -

"Working in the field of mental health, we use humour to ease the strain and to survive," says the lilting voice of New Brunswick nurse Shelby.

Shelby's natural musical ability and sing-song sense of rhythm convey the following events perfectly.

Mr. Ernie Makum was an arthritic gentleman in his eighties. Prior to his admission the best anyone could say was that he was a remarkably miserable gentleman. On the occasion of his first honeymoon, he pushed his wife into a room and nailed the door shut. His first marriage ended. When we attempted to contact his second wife, she refused to respond. His medical history was scant.

This nasty hermit was sent to us because he was so well-known in his area that no nursing home or care facility would take him, based on his reputation. We felt he certainly had been suffering from something, but obviously had never been treated.

The only phrases he ever uttered, other than specific requests, were these words:

"Jumpin' Jesus, jumpin' Jesus, jumpin' Jesus Christ.

Jumpin' Jesus, jumpin' Jesus, jumpin' Jesus Christ."

We heard it so often that we gave the lyrics a little tune. One of my colleagues, while studying the time book, subconsciously rocked from foot to foot, singing:

"Jumpin' Jesus, jumpin' Jesus, jumpin' Jesus Christ.

Jumpin' Jesus, jumpin' Jesus, jumpin' Jesus Christ."

On Monday I had Ernie in the tub room. Now, Ernie could be loud and specific about his needs. We had to fully clothe him, so I had everything there and ready to go — pants, shorts, shirt, socks, shoes.

"MAKE SURE THOSE PANTS GOT PLENTY OF BALL ROOM IN THEM."

"Yes sir. Yes Mr. Makum."

Great gigantic jogging pants for goodness sake that I could put a five hundred pound person into. And boxer shorts, of course, not jockey shorts, because I didn't know where they were going to get caught up. Boxer shorts that belonged to someone at least three sizes larger, but he didn't complain because they gave him BALL ROOM.

I could only get one or two stands from this gentleman because of his severe arthritis, so I layered all the clothing in the right order. While he was sitting, I put his feet into the shorts first and then into the jogging pants.

The plan was simple. When I was ready, he'd stand up while I quickly pulled his shorts and pants up, and he would sit down, his bottom half-dressed. I was ready.

"Would you stand up for me Mr. Makum? One-two-three — Heave."

He stood up. I started pulling on the shorts, started pulling on the jogging pants, and I'm pulling and I'm pulling — and I'm pulling. I only had so many seconds before he couldn't stand any more.

I was pulling, but the shorts and jogging pants were not coming up. What the problem was I could not say.

"I'm awfully sorry Mr. Makum. I'm afraid I'm going to have to get you to sit down again."

"Jumpin' Jesus, Jumpin' Jesus, Jumpin' Jesus Christ.

Jumpin' Jesus, Jumpin' Jesus, Jumpin' Jesus Christ."

The lyrics were getting louder. I had to sort the problem out smartly. The jogging pants were on correctly, but I had put both of his legs into the same leg of the boxer shorts. I could not coordinate the two together up his ass because his legs were as twisted as they were.

"I'm awfully sorry, Mr. Makum, but I'm going to have to ask you to stand again."

"JUMPIN' JESUS CHRIST. WHY?"

"I'm awfully sorry," I said. "I appear to have made a mistake and I had to rearrange your clothing."

"JUMPIN' JESUS CHRIST. WHAT DID YOU DO THAT FOR?"

"What can I say Ernie. I'm incompetent."

"JUMPIN' JESUS CHRIST. YES, YOU DARN WELL ARE!"

By then, of course, I couldn't get another stand out of him and I had to get another nurse to help me. These are the wonders of working in mental health. We love every minute.

THE PANTS
- R - R - R -

"*I started nursing in northern Manitoba after completing various post-graduate university courses,*" says Bridgette. "*I wanted to make a difference.*"

The difference Bridgette made on one particular shift was enough for the RCMP to tease her for many shifts to come.

The regular full-time nurse had gone out on a home visit, leaving me by myself in the clinic, second day on the job. I got a phone call from the RCMP dispatcher saying they were bringing in an abdominal stab wound.

I heard a truck pull up and a door slammed hard. The other nurse was back. Thank heaven. She would handle the case and I would assist.

But it was the RCMP bringing someone in. I have seen people who have been stabbed and they are usually brought in quickly because people panic.

Not so here. This man ambled in behind the RCMP officer, wearing a beautiful white turtleneck sweater and designer jeans. Covered in blood from the waist down.

I took him into the emergency room.

"Get off your pants and get on the stretcher."

My gloved hands trembled ever so slightly as I stood there with a sheet, waiting to cover him up.

"Pardon me?"

"Take off your pants and get on the stretcher."

He looked at the RCMP officer, his eyes pleading for help.

"I said, take your pants off and get up on that stretcher NOW."

With one last imploring glance in the direction of the RCMP officer, he took everything off, ginch and all, and climbed up onto the stretcher. I examined him. No abdominal stab wound.

"You said he was stabbed in the gut," I whispered to the RCMP officer.

"Look, I got a call about a stabbing and this man was covered in blood from the waist down. What does it look like to you?"

Seeking the best source of information, I turned to my patient. "Where are you bleeding from?"

"My right shoulder," he said.

I could hear snickering from the other side of the curtains.

"There's no blood on your sweater. What happened?"

"I changed my sweater," he said.

"Well," I said, "take your sweater off."

He had a small bloody stab wound in his right shoulder requiring eight stitches. I did this as quickly as possible, but I could see he was ticked off for having to take his pants off.

On the way out the RCMP officer winked at me. "I know which nurse I want to see when I cut my shoulder," he said.

Two days later we had a patient who had been severely beaten with chains. The other nurse had him strip to have pictures taken for evidence. She handed me his clothes and said, "Put these in a bag so his family can take them home."

I threw his pants and shirt over my arm and went searching for a clothes bag. Who should I bump into but my friend the RCMP officer. When he saw the pants I was carrying he grinned like a Cheshire cat. My chances of ever living this down are zero.

ODOUR EATERS
- ℞ - ℞ - ℞ -

Ever the discreet nurse who will go to any lengths for her patients, nurse Katy solved a reeking mystery on a surgical floor in Nova Scotia.

We had this elderly gentleman who was a post-operative TURP or trans-urethral resection patient. Whenever we went into his room a foul odour we couldn't identify totally enveloped us. Talk about rank. It almost smelled like a pseudomonas type of odour.

We tried to be discreet. Housekeeping cleaned the room and used all kinds of disinfectants and sprays. We made sure his personal hygiene was beyond reproach. We sent his urine to the lab for tests, thinking maybe he had a urinary tract infection. The results came back negative.

We asked him directly if he smelled anything unusual. No, he said, he didn't smell anything out of the ordinary. We were baffled.

Several odour-eaters later we discovered where the foul smell was coming from. Underneath his clothes, in his locker, was this dried fish he had taken so much care to hide from us.

In the Maritimes there is a scattered population of French Canadians, and one of their traditional delicacies is salted, dried fish. They make it by placing a fresh filleted fish like haddock or cod in a salty brine. In the olden days they used to hang the fish up on lines to dry in the sun, but now they have dryers inside.

Once you've smelled dried fish, you know what it is. It's really rank if you're not used to it, but to our patient this was like caviar and worth guarding with his life.

I purchased a tightly-sealed container to put his fish in, and he always kept it within reach. We were happy the mystery was solved and we didn't have to smell the fish any longer.

COME QUICK, MAID
- R - R - R -

"I was getting to know the area and the hundred and fifty people in my outpost nursing station in Labrador/ Newfoundland."

So began Yolanda's northern nursing adventures.

140

As I was soon to discover, everybody is either aunt, uncle, or skipper over in Labrador, and maid is a common expression referring to any girl. In early September, ten days after getting there, I got a frantic phone call from Aunt Sadie Hannell.

"Come quick, maid. Come quick. Joey's got his throat torn out. He was in a terrible fight. Will you come?"

"Yes, Aunt Sadie. I'm on my way."

I grabbed the little black bag I had in readiness for every possible contingency. Aunt Sadie's house wasn't far from the nurses' station and I went chugging down the dirt path, round the pond, up the bend, through the back door into the house, and on into the back kitchen. I was huffing and puffing, being the athlete that I am. "Okay, I'm here," I panted.

Aunt Sadie had eight children and her family was one of the patriarchal members of the community. They were all there, absolutely hysterical.

"Who's hurt?" I asked.

"It's Joey, maid," Aunt Sadie sobbed. "Joey."

I looked in the direction of her trembling finger. Two of her tallest sons were crouching in the corner. Between them a gigantic German shepherd stood growling, blood splatting down to the floor in big dark drops. The dog's throat had been savagely ripped open by an even larger dog from the other side of the pond.

"That's a dog, Aunt Sadie."

"Oh yes, maid. I'm so glad you're here, you're going to help."

"Aunt Sadie," I said, "what can I do? That's a dog."

"You're the almighty nurse. You can fix him."

I have always been afraid of any dog larger than a teapot. I opened my little black bag and started rocking back and forth, childlike. I didn't know what to do. They're going to know I'm from New Brunswick, I thought.

Right then and there I decided to do something. I looked at the dog's throat and yes, it was in desperate need of stitches. And yes, they did teach me how to do stitches, but they didn't say anything about a dog.

"I'm not going near that dog unless he's laying down," I said. "Out. Sleeping."

What won't kill it might cure it, I thought. What would a veterinarian do if he wanted to get this German shepherd to lay down? I looked around in my black bag at all manner of sedatives.

I drew up 100 mg. of Largactil. The only method I knew of giving an intramuscular injection was into the gluteus muscle in the hip.

I got the two sons to hold the dog while I carefully mapped out the gluteus muscle and shot the sedative in.

"Put the teapot on, Aunt Sadie," I said. "I'm not going near this dog until he's down for the count."

The family, who was never allowed to smoke in Aunt Sadie's kitchen, gave me permission to smoke because they couldn't bear to see me wringing my hands. We sat there drinking tea and watching the dog. Eventually he sat down.

I stood up. The dog stood up.

"I won't touch that dog as long as he's standing up," I said, reaching into my bag. I drew up another 100 mg. of Largactil, and with the help of the two eldest sons, shot it into his other hip.

Within a couple of minutes I felt safe enough to shave an area around the cut on Joey's neck, his doggy breath hot on my quivering hands. I must have poured an entire bottle of hydrogen peroxide into the cut before stitching it up.

I'm a midwife. In obstetrics we use chromic 3 suture, which is heavy as barbed wire and doesn't have to be removed — it absorbs itself. That's what I used on Joey.

I got three good stitches in, leaving a half inch gap. One more stitch and I was out of there.

The dog stood up. I jumped out of the way. "That's perfect," I said. "You see that little gap there, Aunt Sadie? That'll drain out any infection. What I'll do is leave you this other bottle of hydrogen peroxide and get you to wash this area every day. Make that three times a day. And we'll give him some antibiotics. Give him two capsules four times a day. I'll start him off good with an injection now."

Joey didn't much care what I did at this point, groggy as he was. I left him in the good hands of his loving family.

Back at the nursing station we had a log book in which all visits, procedures, and materials used were to be entered for billing purposes. I tallied the cost up in my head, but decided not to make the entry, thinking my supervisor would never understand.

Joey healed well. Aunt Sadie told the story to anyone who would listen. "Look at that," she'd say proudly, pointing to Joey's restored throat. Joey wagged his tail appreciatively.

My supervisor came five weeks later, and I tested the waters by running a variation of Joey's story past her.

"Nurse," she said, "I hope you understand that in this line of work you have to perform many roles, and one of them could be in the area of veterinary science," and she flew back to Newfoundland.

The next time the plane delivered my weekly-cum-monthly vegetable order, there, buried under the carrots and the broccoli, was a thick blue book entitled *Diagnosis and Treatment of Veterinary Science.*

BELGIAN DAINTIES
- ℞ - ℞ - ℞ -

In Nova Scotia, medical nurse Ada says, "We have a four-bed male ward, and one night it was busy as usual. By the end of the evening I had to indulge one of my secret passions to prove a point to my patient."

Sammy, one of the older gentlemen, was a heavy-duty drinker with a kindly heart. His lady friend came to visit, dressed to kill in leopard jacket and black tights, red hair pinned back in an exotic style with a diamond-studded comb. Her expensive perfume wafted through the floor.

As a special gift for Sammy, she brought in a beautifully wrapped box of delicious Belgian chocolates. Delighted, he passed the chocolates around to the three other men in the room, deriving as much pleasure from his generosity as they did. I too indulged in the Belgian dainties. They were nothing short of scrumptious.

The moment of ecstasy was short-lived, however. Five minutes later the elderly man in the bed next to Sammy unexpectedly arrested. We called a code, but despite our best efforts at resuscitation, he died as a result of a long-term heart condition.

After all the commotion settled down, I heard someone moaning and carrying on. I looked over. Sammy was crying.

"What's the matter, Sammy?"

He wiped his tear-streaked face. "I killed that man," he sobbed. "I gave him one of my chocolates."

We couldn't help but laugh at the connection Sammy made. I explained that his friend's heart condition did him in, and to prove my point, polished off the rest of his Belgian chocolates.

145

Lillian R. Tymchuk, RN

THE POTTY AND THE RCMP OFFICER
- ℞ - ℞ - ℞ -

When Verna came in for her nursing duties on the day shift in Prince Edward Island, she found the fears of a young patient mirrored her own.

Margy, a two-year-old patient in diapers, greeted me as I came in to work one morning. I decided we should potty train her and put the potty in the room beside her bed. All day long she did very well, encouraged by her roommate, a pretty five-year-old girl.

Four o'clock come and we were giving report. I told them about the potty training. Before I left for the day, we got a phone call concerning a female overdose who was coming. I still hadn't finished signing off my medications, so I volunteered to stick around in case they needed extra help.

Meanwhile, the LNA who had come on duty saw the potty had been used, covered it, and went to the bathroom to empty it. But somebody was in the bathroom, so she set the potty by the door.

When the RCMP brought the overdose in, the doctor and other nurses performed a gastric lavage on her. She was extremely combative and they were having quite a time. Supper time arrived, so I stayed and passed the trays out, as well as the medications.

One mother had come in to feed her little boy. She happened to be the aunt of Margy's roommate. By then, I was holding one baby in my arms and feeding another in his high chair.

All of a sudden we heard this frightened screaming from the two little girls up the hall. I promptly put the baby into his crib and went to see what the problem was. En route, I saw a handsome, immaculate Mountie standing at the desk. Giving him a curt nod, I hurried to the girls' room.

In the doorway the five-year-old was screaming and crying, pointing to the crisp red uniform. She was scared to death of the Mountie.

Meanwhile, Margy was jumping up and down on her bed, and these little brown turds were coming out from underneath her panties. And I couldn't find the potty anywhere.

The Mountie watched solemnly as I trudged back up to the desk, cradling Margy in my arms. Both of us were covered in turds.

"Would you like to sit in the solarium and I'll get you a cup of tea," I said. I was half scared of Mounties myself.

ROOM FOR HUMOUR
- R - R - R -

"The thirty beds in the new lodge for out-of-town cancer patients was in a separate wing of the hospital. The beautiful brass beds and homey furniture gave it the appearance of a classy hotel. I became the manager there."

Lillian R. Tymchuk, RN

This is nurse Alana's story from Ontario.

I decided to research laughter and to open up a humour room after listening to a presentation by a senior citizen who started the *Laughing Does Matter* group.

Our new lodge had a rarely used music room, so I targeted this area. I got quite a bit of resistance from the director, but I planned to raise money through volunteer groups and donations.

I set up a laughter resource committee comprised of a physician, social worker, two volunteers from the Cancer Centre, two other nurses, and myself.

We each took an aspect of laughter, such as books or videos, as our homework project and we met every month. After a year and a half we had the backup to say yes, laughter was beneficial. Money and donations were generously given by groups such as the Lions Club.

The United States has numerous humour rooms, but because this was something new in Canada we got a wonderful response to our official opening, with lots of hoopla and media attention.

Skeptics wondered what was so funny about having cancer. We showed that if you remove yourself from the situation and take the time to laugh, it's going to help in the long run, because you can't feel depressed and angry and frustrated while you're laughing. It's like taking a recess in your life, a break to regenerate yourself. That was our approach.

Our patients stayed in the lodge five days a week, for up to six weeks, depending on the length of treatment. They came for chemotherapy or radiation, or both. On weekends they either went home or found alternate accommodation.

We didn't impose the humour room on anybody. Some people heard others laughing and decided to join them. Other people chose not to. But I found that in the middle of the night when worried patients woke up, they would often wander down to this room.

An anxious fifty-year-old woman from up north arrived for radiation following a lumpectomy for breast cancer. Her prognosis was fairly good, but she was terrified of radiation because of stories she had heard about what her skin might look like afterward. She half-believed it would glow in the dark.

Following her admission she had several hours to wait before her first treatment. She walked past the humour room where three patients were roaring with laughter at *The Money Pit*, a comedy starring Shelley Long. What's humour got to do with cancer, she wondered.

Nonetheless, she joined the others and stayed to watch John Candy in *Planes, Trains, and Automobiles*, and Bill Cosby. When the time for her treatment came she was laughing out loud.

She said she was in such a jovial mood she didn't care what they did to her. She started joking around with the therapist and was able to get through her first treatment with relative ease. That, for me, was the most vivid example of laughter dissipating fear.

Because of our successes I opened up a humour room in the lodge of another hospital six months later, but we had to be careful how we introduced laughter. We realized that we couldn't approach everybody at such a difficult time — we had to be very sensitive.

We got numerous calls from other hospitals, patients, family members, and caregivers wanting to know how to do what we had done. I get a lot of satisfaction from that.

I'm the founder of National Laughter Day which is on June 21st. That's the first day of summer, and laughter is like a ray of sunshine in your life. It's also the longest day of the year, and I think we need all the laughter we can get. Because National Laughter Day is so close to Canada Day, it can be linked to Canadians having a good time together as a family.

THE DIPLOMAT
- ℞ - ℞ - ℞ -

Alberta nurse Rhonda says, "We used to be in a four- bed ward and then we moved into a brand new burn unit, much to the joy of all the nurses and patients."

Opening day was a proud moment and a particularly exciting one for our staff, as it promised much-needed equipment and supplies. During many months of renovation, we learned to adapt to limited space and to a less than desirable environment to support patient care.

We were leaving our functional nursing station behind, which was in the bathroom of two adjoining bedrooms. Our charting was done on a piece of plywood placed precariously over the toilet, and a snappy red tool cart held our medications, needles, and other supplies.

The cleansing and debriding of burn wounds, as well as dressing changes, could now be done within the unit. Previously the patients were transported by stretcher to the physiotherapy department for wound cleansing, then returned to the unit for dressing application. It was quite uncomfortable.

The unit was to service southern Alberta and the interior of British Columbia, and Saskatchewan if necessary. Many groups of individuals contributed to the successful achievement of a better facility. The unit attracted much attention and many groups arranged an appointment to tour our new burn treatment unit.

On this particular day, the staff gathered as usual and decided the order of patient care and dressing changes. By mid-morning, we were preparing to take Russell, one of our more serious patients, to the hydrotherapy tank for treatment.

After we provided him with analgesics, he was assisted onto the stretcher and we entered the hydrotherapy room. On the four corners of the stretcher frame, under the patient, we attached our hydraulic lifting device. This intelligent piece of equipment not only lifts the patient, but also weighs him. But in order to obtain an accurate weight, the patient is left dangling from the ceiling.

Although Russell had been through the ritual for weeks, he had become septic, and confusion was setting in. After being accused of everything under the sun, we retrieved him and consoled him. It was no fault of his that he did not understand what was going on.

Once over the tub he was gently lowered in, totally in the nude. It's actually a big whirlpool in the shape of a snow angel, and is filled with water, ten litres of salt, and 500 ml. of betadine.

Within the hour he underwent debridement of the old tissue, cleaning of his burn wounds, exercises with the physiotherapist and the occupational therapist, and finally, examination of his wounds by the staff physician and his entourage of interns and residents.

It's no wonder Russell was thoroughly confused and he demanded we call the meeting to order. Fortunately for us, he considered the move from the hydrotherapy tank to the treatment room to be an excellent motion.

In the treatment room we reapplied his burn dressings. He was not too eager to participate in this activity. With his arms flailing, he presented quite a challenge for us to apply the dressings. We soon found gauze, ointments, and creams all around us. It was not the neatest dressing we had ever done, but it covered the wound and that's all that counted. We put polysporin on his facial burns and flamazine from the neck down.

Once Russell was back in his own bed, he found the intravenous and naso-gastric tubes too cumbersome and he removed them. His most recent skin graft was on his back and required him to lie prone.

As we settled him in he began to complain of abdominal discomfort. His abdomen was indeed firm and we realized he had not had a bowel movement for several days. We provided our usual bowel routine, which included giving him a laxative twice a day, but constipation is a problem because of chronic narcotic use.

Consequently we gave Russell a fleet enema. Within minutes he had the smelliest, most explosive results all over the beautiful new wallpaper and all over our gowns. It was terrible, but it was really the most hilarious thing. We could not stop laughing.

With tears streaming down our faces, the last few challenging hours had changed into a memorable day in the life of a burn patient and the staff. It had actually been a terrible two hours. We were so stressed out, but now it didn't seem to matter, because this funny episode somehow made it better.

Precisely at that moment there was a knock at the door. Opening it just a crack, the assistant head nurse explained she was giving some Chinese diplomats a tour of the unit. This was November and the Olympics were coming in February. So we were getting different groups wanting to see the burn unit, like the Flames hockey team and various political groups from other countries.

This Chinese delegation had asked to see us in action with a patient, but there was no bathroom attached to this particular room and there we were, covered in ...! We were in no position to see our best friends, let alone political diplomats.

After a few minutes of small talk the assistant head nurse poked her head in cautiously. With an initial look of disbelief, followed by a knowing look of "I've been there," she closed the door and encouraged the dignitaries to examine other facets of the new unit.

Incidentally, Russell had an excellent recovery. Although he was extensively burned, he did remarkably well. He visits us periodically and is a member of a burn support group that visits other patients who have experienced similar injuries.

THE TURKEY BASTER
- ℞ - ℞ - ℞ -

Always be cautious before accepting a dinner invitation, advises nurse Clare in the Yukon.

A lady who said she had been constipated for several days called seeking help. I went through the usual advice. She said she had used a laxative in the normal dose, without the desired effect, and was becoming quite uncomfortable.

The drug stores were closed. I asked her if she had any suppositories and she said no, she didn't. I suggested she buy a fleet enema at the drug store in the morning.

"I want to do something tonight," she said, "at home. I was thinking of giving myself an enema with my turkey baster."

FIVE

UNEXPECTED BLESSINGS
- ℞ - ℞ - ℞ -

I feel a feeling which I feel you all feel.
Bishop George Ridding, 1828-1904

Registered nurses, like everyone else, feel good about unexpected blessings. In nature these blessings can take the form of unanticipated rainbows after tumultuous thunderstorms, warm summer breezes that airily offer gentle kisses to anyone and everyone, the crisp crunching of pure white snow underfoot on a blustery winter's morning, or the wonder of October's generous gifts wrapped in beautiful red and gold ribbons.

The juxtaposition of the unforeseen and the unimaginable often creates a link that memory will cherish for a lifetime. For instance, imagine pounding the cold hard cement streets of the city when suddenly the strains of Pachelbel's *Canon In D* float by, perfectly executed by an unseen violinist who is practising in a hidden upstairs apartment with the windows open. The unforeseen and the unimaginable.

At work, imagine running your feet off on a particularly difficult and busy shift without time for supper, when suddenly the aroma of a piping hot pepperoni and double cheese pizza comes floating by, a gift from a grateful and observant patient. Better yet, imagine suicide hot chicken wings with extra servings of blue cheese dip. Mmmmmmm. Unexpected blessings indeed. Or the sudden appearance of a dozen fresh doughnuts — preferably with red jam in the centre — that generous ambulance drivers or police officers make the time to bring in.

Sometimes blessings aren't always obvious but all that is required is that each nurse is aware of the present moment. In the beautiful bittersweet stories which follow, the nurses feel blessed in ways that are surprisingly unrelated to daily expectations. The unforeseen and the unimaginable. Carpe Diem.

PICTURE THIS
- R - R - R -

"*I'm a transport nurse,*" explains Janice, one of *10,334 nurses in Manitoba.* "*Sometimes our team members feel like professional paparazzi, because a Polaroid camera is part of our standard equipment.*"

We either fly or drive the ambulance to peripheral hospitals anywhere within a hundred mile radius to bring critically ill patients to major centres where treatment can be enlarged upon. Although I love being a transport nurse, one of the hardest parts is not always being able to follow up on our patients.

The doctor, respiratory therapist, and I flew out for Michael, a newborn baby who developed serious breathing problems and required more sophisticated care.

Michael's skin was a dusky hue and we had to quickly determine whether his heart or lungs were the cause of his distress. We ruled out the lungs, and decided a severe heart defect was causing his problems. He required immediate surgery to correct this defect.

Our magic hour for taking baby pictures is before we insert any tubes or IVs, and Michael was no exception. Afterward we exposed his problem to his parents and obtained a surgical consent. His mother hoped to be discharged soon enough to hot-shoe it over to our hospital with her husband, less than an hour away by car. She wanted to be with her baby.

As we zoomed in for the landing, the surgical team was ready for Michael's imminent surgery. Sometime later I saw his anxious parents in the waiting area of the operating room, ready to blow up on hearing any negative news. His mother was sobbing, grasping the baby's picture tightly in both hands. In her eyes he was the most photogenic baby in the whole world.

The surgery took almost three hours and Michael would no longer require an airbrush to get rid of that dusky colour. The operation was a success.

I just had time to reload a fresh film into the camera when our team got another call to pick up yet another sick baby. Whether or not the infants survive, the glossy picture is a permanent record for infinity, of a sad but lovely vignette.

A CLAP OF THUNDER
- R - R - R -

"This is about a baby that came into our unit and our involvement as staff nurses and the ultimate outcome. We did agonize a fair bit with this baby," admits nurse Louise in British Columbia.

Bonnie was three months old when she was transferred to our pediatric intensive care unit. She was very tiny, with a head of black hair and dark eyes, but it was difficult to see her face because of the tape anchoring her naso-endotracheal tube and feeding tube.

She was born nine weeks early. A breech presentation, she was the second born of twins. The mother had delivered the twins herself, on a ferry, and had done mouth-to-mouth resuscitation on this baby.

Bonnie and her sister were transferred to the special care nursery of our hospital several hours later, and because of their low birth weight and immature lungs, required extensive medical intervention and specialized nursing care.

The first twin progressed well and by about two and a half months of age was ready for discharge. After three months, Bonnie was still extremely unstable and unable to breathe on her own. She came to our unit because of her size and the need for continuing intensive care. Now she was big enough to be cared for in a crib rather than in an incubator.

I introduced myself and some of the staff to the parents the day before her admission to orient them to their daughter's new surroundings. I wanted to prepare them for what they could expect at the time of transfer.

I met a Caucasian mother who was carrying the first-born twin, and an aboriginal father. Accompanying them was a two-year-old daughter and two sons, six and seven years of age — a lovely family.

The nursery staff had told me they had some difficulties in meeting the parents' needs. They wanted to visit all the time and wanted to hold their baby more frequently than was expected.

The physician had permitted the family the use of unorthodox treatment, for example, the use of garlic rubbed on the palms and the soles of the feet, which is an aboriginal tradition. Also the shaman, or holy man, had come in several times and chanted quietly at Bonnie's bedside.

Both parents seemed pleased with their daughter and her move to a pediatric area. They liked the size and the openness of our unit, the toys, the colourful posters on the wall, and they especially appreciated the family unit next door.

I explained that we encourage the family to be there as much as possible and we would involve them in their baby's care. To us, the fragile child, the siblings, and the parents all required our care.

Upon arrival, Bonnie required continuous mechanical ventilation with a rapid ventilatory rate of about sixty a minute, and she was on one hundred percent oxygen. Because of this tube she required one-to-one nursing, frequent suctioning, physiotherapy, and positioning because she could not move on her own, and blood gases every four hours. She was fed by a naso-gastric tube and tolerated small amounts of breast milk, which her mother provided to us several times a day. Like all babies, she needed to be cuddled and stimulated with music and toys and human voices.

We included the parents input in the preparation of the nursing care plan, and this helped us in providing consistency for all shifts. I also met with their social worker, who explained that this was a family of limited financial means.

For the past three months they lived in a motel near the hospital, and the two older children had been placed in public school. But the family planned to stay with Bonnie until she was ready to go home. They had the support of a fairly large aboriginal community, although no close friends or family were here on site.

The social worker said she had discussed the possibility of the baby's death with the mother, but the father was not prepared to discuss it, as it was his aboriginal belief to focus only on the positive.

Within the first few days of the baby's transfer to our unit it was obvious to me how fragile and ill Bonnie was. She required one-to-one care, and two nurses to move her and all her tubes. She was frequently restless and fought against the tubes and the suctioning and the physio, and it was a challenge to prevent her from twisting her head, which could result in the tubes being pulled out. Even with one hundred percent oxygen, her colour would become dusky and her heart rate would drop. The mother had a good understanding of her daughter's condition and of the technical equipment and nursing care supporting the life of her daughter. Both parents asked many questions directly about the blood work, ventilator changes, and medication. We worked hard to be honest and consistent in our answers.

The parents continued their involvement in her care by changing Bonnie, bathing, turning, holding, and settling her with our assistance. They expressed their delight in doing some of the normal things for her.

We took pictures of her when all the tubes and tapes were off during re-intubation. The physician allowed us a few seconds, because babies look so different without everything attached. The pictures gave them a life-long keepsake. I organized the first nursing care conference on Bonnie at the end of the first week and included the physician, other health care personnel, and the parents. The physician saw her daily, but often would not be there when the parents visited. Because of the scope of many of their questions, it was imperative to set some time up with the physician.

At the end of the first month, Bonnie's mother began her wish to start using herbal teas to replace some of the baby's medication. We had a great deal of difficulty with this initially, but she brought in some books for the nurses to look at. She was feeling like many of us, that nothing was helping this baby improve.

Bonnie was unable to absorb breast milk, and I eventually felt comfortable in helping the mother present this idea to the physician. She did the library research about the herbal medicine and at one of our weekly conferences she presented this to him. He was supportive but also cautious, agreeing to read the information and to consult with our pharmacist. Within a week, the mother was bringing in one tea for Bonnie, three times a day. By the end of the third week, she was on three different teas. The staff found this uncomfortable and difficult, a problem we never did resolve. Some teas gave Bonnie gastric distress and diarrhea, and we tried to keep communication open amongst ourselves about this unorthodox treatment.

After a month of receiving these teas, Bonnie was developing more diarrhea and cramps, and a bloated abdomen. Strengths of the teas were varied, but the symptoms persisted and there was a lot of skin breakdown from the stools.

Her condition deteriorated quickly. Her ventilator was at the highest setting possible, and the physician told the parents and staff there was nothing he could do to further improve her ventilation. The chronic changes in her lungs were so severe that adequate gas exchange was not possible. She was more difficult to settle, coughing frequently and moving her head about, in a lot of pain. Unhappily, both medical and nursing interventions frequently inflicted pain upon her, with re-intubation, suctioning, needles, and IVs.

The staff frequently talked about giving Bonnie more sedation, but the mother felt strongly that she not receive too much. She perceived that the baby did not feel as much pain as we indicated, and she was able to settle her most of the time. We worked hard to find an alternative distraction for pain control, such as music, positioning, and toys.

We had several nursing support conferences. We all knew Bonnie was going to die, and it was agonizing to see her suffer every day. Getting together and talking helped us deal with our feelings and to cope with the situation.

I began to worry about the mother. She had used her traditional medicine and yet the baby was not responding. Had we allowed her too much control? We expressed this thought to her, and the physician played his role in determining that he would give the teas one more week and then reassess. At the end of that week the teas were stopped.

With my encouragement, the mother asked the physician for another medical opinion, to be sure everything possible had been done. This was arranged and the conclusion was formed that the baby could not survive and would eventually succumb to infection. The parents accepted this.

The family again met with the staff, physician, and the whole team, and expressed their desire to discontinue treatment and allow Bonnie to have a peaceful death.

As nurses, we had worked hard to respect and facilitate the family's wishes regarding the care of their baby, and to support them once they reached their decision to discontinue treatment.

Several days later the family arrived quite early, accompanied by a shaman. The mother bathed the baby, and all the family members, including the older children, held her. She was given some sedation and the physician discontinued her from the ventilator and manually ventilated her with the resuscitation bag.

The father held her and we carried her outside the hospital into the fresh air. Our hospital is surrounded by farms and fields, in a serene pastoral setting. It had been a long-time wish on the part of the family that Bonnie feel fresh air on her face.

We walked to a small wooded area. Shortly thereafter, the physician removed the endotracheal tube and the family was left alone with their baby. She died peacefully in about five minutes.

The baby never had to go back into the hospital. They had made funeral arrangements and she was carried to the funeral home in a basket her mother had weaved many years ago.

At the time of Bonnie's death, her family said they heard a small clap of thunder, which signified that one of the gods had reached down and received the soul of this precious child.

BREAKING ALL THE RULES
– ℞ – ℞ – ℞ –

"I was going against all the rules," says ICU nurse Eleanor in Nova Scotia, *"but what my patient needed was my special brand of psychological care."*

Hennie, a spunky redheaded seventy-year-old Scottish female who had never been hospitalized before, was admitted to the intensive care unit with a heart attack. She made sure I knew that while she did dye her hair now, she was a true redhead when she was younger.

While Hennie was hospitalized, she discovered she was diabetic and would be required to alter her dietary habits. This poor lady had difficulty in adjusting to her illnesses because she had always been healthy, and it was hard for her to take.

In our unit, we had a central desk with five walled cubicles around the desk, and each cubicle contained one bed. On night shift we worked alone unless we had a patient on a ventilator, and then we had a backup. This meant we ate our meals there because we never got relief for our breaks.

Hennie, in her cubicle, was located about six feet directly behind me. She wasn't a good sleeper. One night I was eating my highly nutritious supper of lasagna and doughnuts when she woke up, and I could tell she wanted to share my meal.

She was booked for a fasting blood test in the morning. I knew I would be breaking all the rules, but in my mind, she needed a treat more than she needed another blood test.

I set up an elaborate, forbidden picnic for the two of us, using a white bedsheet for a tablecloth and one of her floral bouquets as a centrepiece. A bright, new spark ignited in her eyes. As we happily devoured doughnuts and lasagna, she saw that the possibility of fun and laughter still existed for her.

I guess what she liked most was that we were sneaking behind the physician's back and breaking the hospital's rules. Psychological nursing at its best. Needless to say, I accidentally on purpose forgot she was fasting for her test in the morning.

What was funny about it was that she did extremely well from that night forward. Months after her discharge she returned for a visit. She promised me she was complying with her new diet and I had to admit she looked absolutely fabulous, with her flaming red hair and a new gleam in her eye.

After she left I noticed a string-tied parcel on the corner of the desk. Ripping it open, I could smell delicious home-made lasagna and my favourite French crullers. Sometimes rules are meant to be broken.

Lillian R. Tymchuk, RN

THE TEDDY BEAR
- R - R - R -

Sometimes rules are meant to be enforced. At great potential danger to herself, Jeannie, an emergency room nurse in Saskatchewan, made a brave nursing decision to do just that, whatever the cost.

Our ER is laid out like a big square "O" and the inside of the circle is solid. It's remarkably like a square racetrack.

We have electronic doors, the kind that open when somebody steps on the pad outside. I was working nights when such a commotion and racket started near the doors, I couldn't imagine what it could possibly be. I was at the back, about one hundred feet from the front door.

All of a sudden in comes this troop — they weren't Hell's Angels but they definitely were a motorcycle group on their bikes. They roared through the front door, each one looking meaner and tougher than the previous one. All wore sleeveless black leather jackets. Six of them rode their bikes in and began making the circle, around and around.

We have police buttons. All I had to do was knock the phone off the hook and the police would come instantly, but I didn't want a shake-down here with the police if it wasn't necessary. These guys didn't have their guns pulled or their knives drawn, they were just driving their bikes around the ER.

The one I picked out as the probable leader was missing his right sock. After watching them circle around three or four times, I got them stopped and quieted down. There was just myself and the doctor there.

We asked them what they were doing here. One of them said somebody had pitched a beer bottle at their leader in one of the bars and hit him on the head. The leader pulled off his helmet, and underneath was a blood-spattered sock, roosting on top of a gaping cut. He was the big tough Joe I had picked out as the probable leader. "You have two choices," I said to the group. "First choice is, get your bikes the hell outside and then you can come back and sit in the lobby. Second choice is, you can wait outside. One or the other. These are the rules."

One by one they drove their bikes out and meekly returned to the waiting room. In the suture room, the leader was the biggest suck you ever saw in your life. He groaned and moaned and begged to have his best friend come in with him. I wondered if it was only for moral support, but he did have an alternative motive. He stuffed his blood-drenched sock into his friend's hip pocket.

The doctor said, "Do you want freezing or not?"

The macho ones usually say, "No, I don't need that," but he wanted the freezing, big pussycat that he was.

Two days later he came in and brought me the cutest teddy bear I ever saw. His motorbike was parked outside.

ORGAN DONATION
- ℞ - ℞ - ℞ -

"I was asked to speak to a family in the intensive care unit regarding consent for organ donation," explains nurse Penny in Alberta. "The physician usually approaches them, but he asked me to do this one because he didn't think the family would consent."

This concerns a twenty-year-old Inuit man from the Northwest Territories who had been brought down to ICU. His mother, Estelle, was with him.

Organ donation is a foreign idea for most of the Inuit who come to our modern hospital. The level of activity in the ICU where her son was must have been frightening for her.

I went to the bedside and spoke with his nurse. Her concern was that Estelle would never understand what this was all about, and I wanted her to know that what I was offering was without any pressure from the hospital. Also for us, it had to be something she really wanted to do, something meaningful.

I invited Estelle and the nurse into the quiet room. I explained who I was, that the other nurse was there as her friend, to help her understand that the discussion was going to be around something she might want to do.

The whole discussion took close to an hour, but the dialogue probably took only a few minutes. There were many long pauses.

There was some preamble to ensure that she could understand me. I spoke slowly and directly to her. She was able to tell me what happened regarding her son's accident and that she had only arrived on the unit that afternoon. The doctors told her that her son — she called him "my boy" — would not live.

She looked down as I was speaking to her. I explained what brain death was. As a result of the accident, her son's brain had swollen so much there was no more blood feeding his brain, and without nutrition and oxygen his brain had died and consequently his body would die.

A shoe made a good example. If you hurt your foot badly, it swells but you can take your shoe off. The swelling will continue but the circulation stays intact. But with a bad head injury, the skull prevents the swelling from going external, and as the pressure comes on the brain, the brain dies.

I told her the machines were keeping her boy alive by providing oxygen, and as soon as the machines were turned off his heart would stop beating. She was sobbing quietly after she got the gist of my explanation.

And then I had the difficult challenge of talking to her about organ donation. I put it to her that when these sad things happen, many people here where we live consider organ donation. Although her son was dead, his organs were still alive — his heart, lungs, and kidneys. There are other people, I said, whose organs have died and their body is still alive.

For organ donation to happen, a patient like her son would have to have an operation in the operating room, and his heart, lungs, and kidneys would be taken from his body. His body would be closed without his own organs, and without the organs of the recipient. This was important, because I was not sure of their belief in burying the body whole, and also I wasn't aware of her level of understanding of organ transplants.

She nodded her head. "If you want to consider organ donation," I said, "your boy could donate his organs, but you should only do this if you feel this is the right thing for you."

She bowed her head down low.

"How would your people feel about organ donation?" I asked.

Although I hadn't planned on asking this question, it was probably the most valuable thing I did, because it took the responsibility of the decision off her — how she would envisage this in her culture. Estelle shook her head. She didn't know. She looked at the ceiling, mumbled in her native language, took a Kleenex and cried. I think she was attempting to communicate with her people through her spirit. Other than her sobbing, the room was deathly quiet. Unlike the other nurse, I did not feel uncomfortable. I felt Estelle was processing her thoughts and feelings.

After about fifteen minutes she said, "I don't know what my people would think about organ donation and taking my boy's heart to save someone else's life. But where I come from, we must always help to save another man's life."

She told me the story of how her husband and brother saved a fisherman who had fallen through the ice into freezing waters. Because they value human life, they were willing to risk their own lives.

"But I don't know what my people would think of organ donation," she said, and once more mumbled in her native tongue and stared at the ceiling. From the tone of her voice I thought she was trying to reach out for guidance.

After a while, she nodded. "Yes, this is right," she said. "If my boy can save someone else's life with his organs, he must do that." She signed the organ donor card.

Tears were pouring down her face by this time. We felt she had gone through a process, and reached a conclusion she felt comfortable with. In the end she said, "I think my people would think it was okay for my boy to be an organ donor."

I offered her the opportunity to talk to somebody, like a native elder, even though I wasn't sure how I would do that — probably I would get hold of a nursing station somewhere. But she just wanted to get home. She seemed very much at peace in making the decision.

As a result of this experience I developed a program for donor family support, based on the health promotion concept of a supportive environment, including the aspect of providing information cross-culturally. I've also written a booklet for donor families called *Opening A Window For Your Grief*.

Within this model, we have a community support group of donor families interacting with other donor families. As a result, we have changed our consent form to include information about special care of the donor's body.

Because of the Human Tissue Gift Act regarding confidentiality, we can't disclose too much, but we do send a letter to donor families indicating where the organs were transplanted, and the age and sex of the recipient.

Another thing that's important to donor families is to receive anonymous acknowledgment from recipients, saying how grateful they are for their gift of a heart or a liver or a kidney. Only in about thirty percent of transplant organs is there an acknowledgment. We're working on one hundred percent. These letters come through us to make sure no names or addresses are included.

This work is rewarding and exciting, and is desperately needed. I often think of Estelle and her decision.

Nurse, Hear You, Hear Me

THE GIFT
- R - R - R -

"Once, when I used to relieve in the outpost nursing stations in the Northwest Territories," nurse Joanne relates, "the Anglican minister in the far north asked me to fly up for the day."

When I arrived, I saw Inuit people running along the edge of a steep cliff. They were shooting at caribou with bows and arrows and they hit one, but it continued running. Quickly, they moved in for the kill.

Hours later, I told the nurses there I would take call for the night, giving them a much needed break. Just before midnight the doorbell rang. Propped in the doorway by a friend was a tall Inuit man who looked sick and shivery. His appearance shocked even me.

He was covered with a caribou hide and a big furry thing perched on his head. Blood dripped down the full length of his body, making him look like a hungry werewolf.

His name was Tiimu. He was part of the group chasing the wounded caribou in the afternoon. They killed it, gutted and cleaned it, and took the furs. In the intensity of the chase Tiimu had thrown his own jacket off.

Later in the day the temperature dropped sharply. They rowed ten chilly miles across the lake, and Tiimu covered his body with the caribou fur. The belly fur he put on his head.

I couldn't get a temperature to register — he was hypothermic. His friend helped me lower him into the tub and we gradually warmed him up. Somebody else notified his wife.

When I was leaving to come back home, who should be at the airport but Tiimu, holding a big beautiful Arctic char for me.

A PLACE OF HONOUR
- R - R - R -

"Everybody was whispering and pointing at me when I walked in. 'That's the nurse ... that's the nurse.'"

So began a wintry afternoon that neo-natal nurse Jane, in Alberta, would never forget."

When the baby for whom I had been primary nurse died, I felt compelled to attend her funeral, an aboriginal one. Joanne, another nurse, accompanied me to the parents' home where the service was being held.

All the furniture had been removed from the living room except a couch where the immediate family was sitting. Gray folding chairs occupied the rest of the room.

The baby's open coffin was at one end of the living room, with one chair beside it, facing everyone else. When I greeted the parents, they asked me if I would sit in the chair beside the coffin. This was the place of honour.

"Would you mind if I sit in the front row?" I asked. "I would feel more comfortable." They said okay.

Two ministers officiated. The one who played the guitar was drunk or certainly under the influence. As he led us in singing *Amazing Grace*, he got into such coughing fits that we all stopped until he composed himself. Each time, however, he started back at the beginning instead of continuing on. We sang *Amazing Grace* for quite some time.

The service dragged to completion and we drove to the cemetery for the interment. "Tessie," Joanne screamed at me. "Stop." I slammed on my brakes.

"I think you're driving on a grave."

Sure enough, I had driven the car right over top of a grave. It was the dead of winter and the graves weren't marked. They were in a field and there were some plastic flowers here, and some holes dug by animals there. I could see the aboriginals did not bury their dead in cement containers, only in coffins. I drove past the other cars and walked over to the family.

After the service was over the tribespeople lowered the coffin down themselves. The coffin was like one of those white styrofoam picnic baskets — it didn't have any clamps to hold the lid on.

One leader managed to get his rope tangled, while the other leader continued releasing his. I was afraid the baby's body would tumble out because the coffin was so sharply angled. I wondered what we would do if that happened, but in due time they got both ropes down and lowered the coffin into the hole.

The grandmother presented me with a beautiful pair of beaded moccasins to thank me for looking after the baby. The events of the afternoon were mollified by her selfless, emotionally charged gesture, and provided a gracious ending to the burial of a sweet infant.

EASTER SUNDAY
- R - R - R -

"This particular pilot and I had flown together many times in the Northwest Territories," explains nurse Tammy, "and this Easter Sunday he and I were flying way up north to pick up a patient who was in labour."

"How come every time I see you," the pilot said, "something happens?"

Despite his comments the flight over was smooth and uneventful. The sun shone brightly and the view was spectacular.

We loaded our patient into the plane and took off. At one thousand feet, I was getting myself organized when my patient's water broke. The baby arrived in a big hurry, and I swear she had a look of anticipatory glee on her tiny red face. I wrapped her in my parka.

The sky started becoming darker and more threatening with each passing moment. All of a sudden we flew into a black cloud and the plane shook all over.

Sparks were shooting everywhere. There was no noise but the lights went out, and I thought we must have collided with another plane. But no other planes were in sight — we had been struck by lightning. The fuselage was burned, but at least the instruments didn't go out.

We made an emergency landing. Our pilot told the ground crew that something always happens with "this nurse." Shaken, he thought this experience a bit extreme, even for me. They checked out the plane, replaced the lights, and on we went, the four of us, on Easter Sunday.

FISH CAKES
- ℞ - ℞ - ℞ -

"It's amazing the things nurses know that may be hidden from ourselves, deep in our subconscious," says nurse Belle in Labrador/Newfoundland. "No one could put a scientific theory to them — they come from experience."

I was the nurse in a one-nurse station in Labrador, where no one could be admitted overnight for quite a logical reason. I had normal duties in the day time from Monday to Friday, so if someone had to stay overnight, there was no one to relieve me.

In my little community there were two or three asthmatic children. When they had acute asthma the parents were distraught. To assist them, I would bring the child into my clinic overnight, even though I was by myself. The closest two-nurse nursing stations were thirty-six miles down the coast either way.

Wally was a little five-year-old from an outside island. His family lived in a shack because their home had burned down in a fire the summer before I came. They had no means to rebuild themselves, and were waiting for the welfare people to cough up some money. It was not a short wait.

The conditions in the home were not amenable to Wally's illness. "Bring him in," I told them. "I'll keep him in the clinic overnight."

What I had there, which was unusual, was a croup tent. I recalled using these tents before with good results whenever we had youngsters with respiratory problems.

Wally had a temperature. I started him on antibiotics and Tylenol, but somehow I felt this croup tent was going to help him. I didn't know what else to do either, so I decided to use it. Hank, the maintenance man, was able to supply compressed air for the tent, but I still needed ice.

It was winter. All Hank had to do was get a fifty pound bucket from salt beef, and fill it up with chopped ice. He placed it on the steps outside the clinic door. From there, I hunked off a chunk with the ax, and stuck it in the back of the croup tent. Very good. I put a sleeping bag on the floor beside Wally's bed, hoping to get some sleep before the next day's clinic.

Wally slept. I tylenoled him, gave him his antibiotics, and set my alarm clock for his next dose at 4:00 A.M.

At four I repeated the process. The ice was gone from the croup tent so I went outside for more, but there was none. I had used it all up. Hank said he got it from the pond, maybe a hundred yards from the clinic.

I made sure Wally was sound asleep before I grabbed my axe and the fifty pound bucket and fired up the snowmobile. I came from the city in New Brunswick, and didn't know how to drive a car, let alone a snowmobile. And I was used to the luxury of electricity and street lights.

It was pitch black, save for the beam from a trusty Eveready flashlight. I hacked at the ice until the bucket was full, stuck it between my legs, and drove back. Inside, I threw some large hunks into the croup tent, and wearily climbed into my sleeping bag.

All too soon, I heard, "Mrs. Nur-rse. Mrs. Nur-rse."

I tried to wake up.

"Mrs. Nur-rse. Mrs. Nur-rse."

"Yes, Wally, yes." I peeled out of the sleeping bag, put the side of the crib down, and opened the croup tent. Wally was a smiling, healthy boy.

"How are you today?" I asked.

"I want breakfast, Mrs. Nur-rse."

"All right," I replied, taking him into the kitchen. "What would you like?"

"Fish cakes."

"Fish cakes? I've got corn flakes, I've got porridge, I think there's a box of rice ... fish cakes? To tell you the truth dear, I don't know how to make fish cakes."

MAKING A DIFFERENCE
– ℞ – ℞ – ℞ –

"Had I not noticed how ill my patient had become," says nurse Samantha in Saskatchewan, *"he would have died alone upstairs. There are times you go home feeling you've made a difference."*

Obie was an old man who had been hospitalized in a small town for eight days with pain in his right side. It refused to budge. He had intravenous and medication for pain, but no tests were done.

When he was transferred to us his temperature was substantially elevated. But he was talkative and very jovial, with only slight abdominal discomfort, when the surgeon saw him. He didn't look distressed and his colour was good. There wasn't much besides the fever to suggest he was unwell.

The surgeon said he would take him to the operating room for an exploratory laparotomy. I prepared him for the OR, even though he was being admitted to the floor first.

While giving Obie three different antibiotics, I observed that he was becoming sweaty and pale. His blood pressure and pulse remained stable, but I attached him to the cardiac monitor and did another EKG. He complained about more abdominal pain, and I phoned the surgeon.

"I know Obie's going to go to the OR," I said, "but I think he needs something for pain now."

The surgeon said, "He looked all right when I was there."

"He's diaphoretic now and his colour is worse," I said. "I have the feeling he's more uncomfortable than he's letting on."

He ordered IV Demerol and Gravol, but it never touched him. His pulse started to creep up, although his pressure remained constant.

I called the surgeon again. "I'm really concerned. I think something's going to happen if you don't get him to the OR right now."

"We have a Triple-A (abdominal aortic aneurysm) coming in. The OR's on hold for her," he reminded me.

"According to last report, she's stable. You could get this man in before she arrives."

"Let's hold off," he said.

The Triple-A was perfectly stable when she arrived. I called the surgeon once more. "This man has to get to the OR now."

"I'll have my resident take a look at him," he said. At least he didn't brush me off. He sent the resident down to examine him. By now Obie was so sweaty I could barely keep the leads from the cardiac monitor on him.

I started another IV. The resident felt Obie probably had perforated his bowel. Within minutes he was in the OR.

The family was upset and crying and I felt badly for them. They would never know what happened, but I felt good about my intervention because I know what the alternative would have been. Obie's operation was a success.

THE UN-BIRTHDAY PRESENT
- ℞ - ℞ - ℞ -

"You get little rewards every now and then," says nurse Libby in Alberta. *"Many of the babies we care for are no bigger than a minute, because they come into this world well ahead of time."*

I think each nurse learns what she can handle as far as primary nursing is concerned — we look after the same babies and families every time we're on duty, maybe for four or five months. If the ending isn't a good one, it's upsetting.

Twice I got too involved, and when those babies died I felt like my own baby had died. I went to both funerals. The last one was out of town, and I was the only nurse who went from here.

Actually the death was quite unexpected. We had the Calgary Stampede in two weeks, and I had bought Ronnie a tiny little cowboy hat that would have fit him perfectly.

I thought he could wear it as a joke while he was laying in bed, but he died unexpectedly a few days before Stampede started.

I didn't know what to do with the hat — I certainly didn't want to upset his family. I walked into the church carrying this cowboy hat, thinking maybe there was a place I could put it beside the coffin. No one needed to know it was me who brought it. But there was no coffin at the front, just Ronnie's picture.

I carefully placed it beside me on the church pew during the service. Afterward, when the family called me over to their car, I presented it to them. Everyone passed it around, and it was a smashing hit for the rest of the day. Such little rewards are a real bonus and very meaningful to us.

JAMES' BOND
- ℞ - ℞ - ℞ -

"My most valuable nursing experience so far was on the cardiology service," says a delighted nurse Melody in British Columbia. *"The love of an infant infiltrated my whole being."*

185

James, a newborn, was admitted to the isolation area on the cardiac floor with multiple heart defects. We used this area for kids who were sicker than the rest, and that certainly was James.

From the moment I spied him, peeking from under his covers, I knew something was different. There was immediate bonding. It wasn't as though he was the cutest or most gorgeous baby; actually, his skin was bluish. Perhaps it was his intelligence, I don't know.

He had an emergency shunt and heart repair done, but he was far from stable. His parents were calm, reflective, and down-to-earth people, with three other kids at home.

I was his primary nurse for one week, during which many investigations were done. When his lab reports and test results returned, the doctors decided to send him home. There was nothing more that could be done for him.

In ten years of nursing I had never been more upset. I've cared for many babies with serious heart problems and held my emotions in check, managing difficult situations with professional self-control. I saw many babies die. Now, for some unknown reason, I detected a difference.

The family informed me they were taking James to another hospital for palliative care. When I got home from work that night I found myself thinking about them and, not knowing if it was professional or not, I called the other hospital.

"When the parents of this baby arrive," I said to the receiving nurse, "please tell them that I'm thinking about them." That was the extent of it.

Three weeks later I received some mail from the parents. James had died. I don't know how they uncovered my home address, but they enclosed several snapshots, and a letter saying how appreciative they were of my care. We didn't stay in touch after that. Case closed.

A year later I was working on the dialysis unit. "There's someone downstairs to see you," one of my friends said furtively.

"Who is it?"

"Do I have 'tattletale' stamped on my forehead? It's a surprise."

It was James' family, squealing with delight over their brand new, healthy, baby girl. I have yet to understand why our bond was so strong, but James' memory shines in a secret section of my heart.

A DIAMOND IN THE ROUGH
- ℞ - ℞ - ℞ -

"When I was working on an acute psychiatric floor in Prince Edward Island," explains nurse Elizabeth, "I met a disturbed patient who made me thankful I had the opportunity to meet her."

We admitted Joan, a psychotic forty-five-year-old lady to our floor. She constantly used word association. Colours and numbers, especially the number nine, were important to her.

Joan had had a horrendous life. She had grown up in PEI before moving out west. She had been sexually abused as a child and her marriage was rife with physical and sexual abuse. She had five children before returning to the island, and eventually divorced her husband.

When she came back the RCMP had to admit her. They were concerned for her safety and took her to emergency where she was examined and found to be psychotic.

She was a big woman, rough and tough on the outside. If someone saw her on the street they'd probably turn away. But she was someone I liked immediately and connected with on some higher level. In spite of her gruffness, I felt she projected warmth.

She did get better, but a delusion continued to haunt her. It concerned a man she said she had met out west and she was always looking for him.

When I worked in the community, she was referred to me as a client on welfare. At that time she used drugs, drank, and became depressed enough to want to die, but her Catholicism prevented her from harming herself. She was coarse but there was something sweet about her too.

She moved into a boarding house where each person had their own room. If any of the other tenants were short of money she'd help them out. Sometimes she'd get the money back and sometimes she wouldn't.

Through all this she kept looking for this man, thinking she saw him here and there. In the rest of her life, she functioned well enough. If she didn't talk about him, nobody would know. Eventually she stopped drinking and came off drugs.

It would take me a million years to live through all the stories she used to tell. To her, this was life. "Look at all the stress you've had," I'd tell her, "and you lived through so much, and you're still such a good person."

On welfare, there isn't much money for clothes. At Christmas I'd always get her a gift because she felt so good if she had something nice to wear.

She never thought she was as good as other people but she gave so much to others. I met a couple of her daughters when they were home and that's what I told them. And they did come to love her again.

She didn't keep in regular contact with her children because their lives were also difficult. In the five years I knew her she got in touch with each of them. They came down to the island and she went out west to see them. But she was depressed and often I wondered if I would see her again.

Once Joan went swimming with a friend and nearly drowned. She realized then how much she wanted to live. She had two or three good years, as good as she could, then went out west to visit her family.

Her children had all been reunited and they came to understand why their lives were the way they were.

One day I got a call from one of her daughters. Joan died of a heart attack. I was thankful it was quick and that she didn't suffer. Life is such an irony.

IT'S NOT WHAT YOU SAY
- R - R - R -

"In communicating, it's not always what you say but rather how you listen that is more important." This is how *Alberta nurse Jean explained an unusual and important experience in her nursing career.*

A twenty-four-year-old man named Bertie came in after being assaulted with a hammer. He was slightly mentally handicapped, and with the new brain injury on top of it, he was in big trouble. He was in a coma for a long time.

For some reason his family, and his mother in particular, saw me as the one person they could always come to and ask questions. His mother felt I always gave her a "straight answer," as she put it.

If the doctor was coming to talk to them about something she would ask him to wait until I could be there. Or if the family couldn't be there for some reason or other, she would ask me to find out what the doctor had to say, and then tell them about it.

Bertie was with us for several months. He was in Intensive Care and back to us, back and forth. In that time, the family and the patient himself strongly identified with the nurses on our unit, and it was like coming home every time he returned to us.

In the course of his recovery, Bertie was transferred to the rehabilitation unit of another hospital, where he stayed for several months. Every time something happened there his mother phoned me to get my perspective. Usually all I was doing was listening to her, and sensing and feeling, finding out what she wanted to do, bolstering or strengthening her, or giving her another outlook.

Bertie is currently in a nursing home. He has recovered reasonably well from his traumatic injury, although not enough to live as independently as before. However, he is cognizant of everything around him.

Almost two years later Bertie's mother still calls me. I can't identify any one special thing I did, but this family always felt they could trust my judgment. This experience reinforced the importance of a trusting relationship, and of keeping communication lines open. And for me, it reaffirmed nursing.

Lillian R. Tymchuk, RN

PRUNE BELLY
- R - R - R -

Pediatric nurses, like Martha in British Columbia, get rewards in subtle, unfathomable ways that leave the recipient's heart dancing.

For some time now nursing had been getting me down. I made a decision to leave nursing and go into computer work full time. Until today, that is.

After a few days off I started day shift on my customary pediatric nephrology floor. I always transform my uniforms into gorgeous, glittery garb, by gluing on a glob of sparkles here, sewing a red heart on there. I like dressing like this because the glitz distracts many kids when they most need it.

Randy is an eight-year-old who only weighs eighteen kilos, so he could be taken for a kid half his age. This gives a good idea of the size of our kids.

Randy has Prune Belly Syndrome. If you think of a prune, you can picture what this kid looks like. His abdominal wall is not firm tissue, it's really wobbly, and his organs are just sitting there. If you look at his tummy, it's all rollie and dented looking. His organs are damaged and he has bowel and kidney problems. This is a congenital condition, but he's made it so far.

When I went in today after being off for a few days, Randy came running up to me, threw his little arms around me, and said, "I missed you."

Computer work wouldn't be the same.

SIX

TRAGEDY - ACCEPTING THE INEVITABLE
- ℞ - ℞ - ℞ -

The bad end unhappily, the good unluckily.
That is what tragedy means.

Tom Stoppard, 1937-

Who said it has to be dark before you can see the stars?

Tragedy often involves betrayal of considerable magnitude, by a person, an ill-held ideal, or both. On the large scale, political and economic forces play havoc in the lives of people who have little or no control over these happenings. They can only control their reactions, but that is easier said than done.

Tragedy moves unwilling participants from one extreme to another with devastating, disastrous, and irreversible results — robust health to paralyzing infirmity, financial independence to total ruin, loving relationships to barren loneliness.

Close observation shows tragedy often compounds upon tragedy. A nurse from Alberta says, "A high percentage of our car accidents are the result of people who have been driving all night to get to a funeral or to the bedside of someone who is ill, and there's a fatality because somebody fell asleep at the wheel." Tragedy compounded upon tragedy.

Personal tragedies become part of the public domain when the enormity of the events becomes so overwhelming as to impact society at large.

How do Canadian nurses contend with the ever-changing yet ever-constant face of tragedy? By looking for the stars.

MY BROTHER'S KEEPER
- ℞ - ℞ - ℞ -

Nurse Renee is one of 64,093 nurses in Quebec. Working in the northern part of her province, she had not only her patients to attend to, she also had a colleague who desperately needed her professional help.

I came back from holidays to discover I would be working with a new colleague named Charmaine. She was a young nurse on the move, extremely active. Hyper, really. I told myself I would need at least a gallon of Geritol to maintain her speed, even though I'm pretty fast myself.

As the week progressed — it was Holy Week — I began to have nagging doubts about Charmaine's behaviour, doubts which were confirmed when her sister called from the south.

"Charmaine never sleeps," she said. "She's always on a high. I'm worried about her."

One night I heard the Inuit say, "Nurse, don't go too far. Come back." In the light of a full moon, Charmaine was wading in the cold waters of a dark river. She emerged fully clothed, dripping wet, and ran full-tilt along the water's edge, circling back to her house. The situation was becoming untenable, dangerous even.

In the days that followed she became more hyper. As president of the union she was making arrangements for a meeting. I called the doctor and he said I must not allow her to go anywhere. I told her the meeting was cancelled.

Her house was a stone's throw away from mine, and I did my best to keep an eye on her. Every night the lights in her house flickered brightly, regardless of the hour, and I could see her dark, animated shadow flit from one window to the next.

When Charmaine's sister called again, I advised her to call the medical director to discuss Charmaine's past medical history. This was on Holy Friday. On Holy Saturday morning the doctor called in. "You'll have to observe your colleague until we can medi-vac her down south," he said.

I decided not to tell Charmaine. There are no police here and because it was a perfect sunny weekend, everyone was out fishing. No one would be available to help me.

I was on call. Two kids had high temperatures and there were the usual injuries. I ran back and forth between the nursing station and Charmaine's house, looking after my patients, and trying to observe Charmaine unobtrusively at the same time.

The doctor called again with details of the medi-vac. I told Charmaine the union meeting had been rescheduled and she could go after all. She was flabbergasted.

"How did you manage that?"

"There's a medi-vac that needs an escort," I said, "so you can go. And a replacement is coming, so you don't have to worry about anything here."

At three in the afternoon I took Charmaine to the airport. She was now the union president. She spread numerous files on the floor and shuffled papers from one pile to another, never getting them quite to her liking. The tense wait was heightened because no one else was around.

I knew there was trouble when a nervous air agent called me aside. The plane, he said, had to overshoot because of two consecutive emergencies. First, a pregnant lady from Frobisher delivered her baby on the plane, but the baby died and they returned to Frobisher. On their way back, they picked up an old man in the next village and he arrested in the air, so they overshot again.

"Is the meeting cancelled?" asked an anxious Charmaine.

We returned to the nursing station. Within seconds, the doctor called. "We're coming back at ten tonight, so have your colleague ready to fly."

In the interim, I suggested Charmaine pack lots of food to take to the union meeting. "Maybe you won't be back next week because of the weather. You never know," I said.

She obeyed because she trusted me. As she finished packing her food she presented me with a delicious maple syrup lollipop, a favourite among my favourites. I sucked on it and rolled it around on my tongue, savouring its sweetness. Hating to think it could be dwindling in size, I removed it from my mouth to see how much was left — and the gleaming bridge from my front teeth came along, tightly clamped onto the lollipop.

"Thee what happened, Tharmaine," I lisped.

She roared with laughter. "We're having a party," she said. Her face was flushed.

The phone rang. It was the doctor. "Tell your colleague she's the one who's going to be medi-vacced," he instructed me.

"Thee trusth me," I replied. "I thuggetht you tell her on the plane. I don't want to upthet her."

A brief moment of silence. "Are you okay?" he asked.

"Yeth," I said, "conthidering the thituation, ith all thettling down nithely."

Just before ten o'clock we arrived at the airport. I escorted Charmaine onto the plane and left her in the care of the doctor.

In the back of the plane I could see one of our stretchers from a previous medi-vac.

"Thath my threther," I said to the pilot. "Thend it down the thepth to me, and I'll thend it back to the nurthing thathion."

He ignored me. He must have thought I was the nurse with the mental problem.

On Holy Sunday I packed up everything from Charmaine's house. While I was there she called me from the hospital, demanding to know why I had medi-vacced her out.

Charmaine refused to take her Lithium while she was hospitalized. She never came back.

SHIFT FROM HELL
- R - R - R -

Nurse Paige shares the acute pain and anguish she encountered during a "shift from Hell" in a busy Saskatchewan trauma centre.

There had been nothing but terrible car accidents for the last several weeks, and it was only the middle of summer.

One weekend we were pre-warned about a fifteen-year-old female, possible head injury, who was being transferred from an out-of-town facility with volunteer ambulance staff.

The dispatcher told us the bike she was riding was struck by a car. She hit her head and there was grave concern about her potential injuries. We were told to page the resident upon her arrival.

When she came in she was sitting on a wooden back board with a Philadelphia collar on her neck, unrestrained. She had no intravenous.

We moved her over to our stretcher and tried to restrain her because she was an obvious head injury. There was some bleeding on her forehead but we weren't sure where it was coming from. We figured she probably would have been about a twelve or thirteen on the Glasgow Coma Scale.

We told her our concerns about her neck, that if she had a fracture there she could end up paralyzed, but we weren't getting through to her. She was making screaming noises, not actually talking or saying words. We decided she was in a state where she could injure herself.

We hooked her up to our monitor. There were three residents present. All of her systems seemed to be fine at the time. She was in normal sinus rhythm on the cardiac monitor, she was breathing on her own, and she was moving her arms and legs well.

We followed our standard trauma procedure and started two large bore IVs of ringer's lactate. She needed to be re-assessed and to have a cat scan (CT) done. Our standard was to do CT heads as quickly as possible, and

CT abdomens when our patients were unable to tell us whether they had pain or any other finding there.

Normally at this point we gave the drugs Valium and Succinylcholine, which we alternated to put these patients under, so we could control them and consequently work more effectively. This had worked extremely well for us in the past.

Consequently we gave these medications IV to this young girl to protect her C-spine and to do a better assessment. However, we were unable to intubate her, for whatever reason, even with the respiratory technician and three residents present.

We bagged her for a while and tried to intubate, bagged and tried to intubate, until this became very traumatic. Everybody was getting more and more concerned and we eventually called the surgeons and the anesthetists to come down and get her intubated.

In this time she arrested. Fifteen years old. A full cardiac arrest.

The anesthetist easily intubated her; the e-tube went in like nothing. We followed the ACLS protocol (Advanced Life Support) to get her heart re-started, and gave Epinephrine and Sodium Bicarb while doing CPR. All of us felt a sense of panic when her monitor was in asystole and we weren't getting anywhere. The next step was obvious.

One of the surgeons grabbed a thoracotomy tray, pierced her chest, and performed open heart massage. We injected intracardiac epinephrine until her heart was able to keep going on its own. In time she reverted to normal sinus rhythm, and was actually doing quite well. We sewed her chest up. Things were stabilizing.

We put her on the little respirator that we keep in Emergency. Our panic level was gradually subsiding. Then we checked her pupils. They were fixed and dilated. This result, even with a full staff of cardiovascular and trauma surgeons.

We did a chest x-ray. There was evidence she had aspirated. No one knew at that time whether this happened during the attempts at intubation or whether she had vomited at some point during the initial head injury.

The CT scan of her head was normal. C-spines, everything ended up being normal, except for this aspirate found in her lung, and the fact that her pupils were fixed and dilated — and she'd had her chest opened up.

From the CT room, we took her to ICU and she was put on a ventilator there. She died two days later. We weren't able to use her organs for donation because she had already been a code. There was absolutely nothing left after that.

Hers was a useless death. It was the only time, in all these years, that I thought we really let somebody down. It was awful. There was a lawsuit. In the haste of the residents wanting to give the Succinylcholine and the Valium like we had always done, perhaps we could have waited until everybody was present and accounted for before going ahead. Had we to do it all over again this girl would be a young lady now.

Even though I was there I have to say I feel it was our fault. There's so much that should have been done differently, but I wasn't prepared to stand up and say, "I think you should wait." Since then, I have always been able to vocalize my concerns.

On the other hand, to be perfectly honest, it was one of those days. We had a young boy with two broken legs, and another man who almost ripped his penis off in a vacuum cleaner. There were only three nurses dealing with all of this.

Perhaps if the staffing had been better, if there had been time to monitor only one patient rather than having our minds on watching hallways and answering phones, the outcome could have been altered.

Had I been more experienced and been through as much as I have now, I wouldn't feel afraid to say, "This is not what needs to be done and I will not be responsible ..." That by itself would have been enough to make them think and to stop.

Sometimes when nurses push doctors into a corner they will go the other way to prove a point. We can tactfully make suggestions to some doctors, but not to others. Residents especially will say, "You're the nurse, but I am the doctor." And sometimes they have it in their heads, "What does she know? She just works here."

After we took the fifteen-year-old to ICU, it was right back to more major trauma. Another young girl with a penetrating wound to the abdomen had to go to the OR, followed by a man with second and third degree burns to sixty percent of his body.

There was no debriefing. We're told that we can call the social worker, but none of us is going to actually step forward and call. I find we debrief in our own way. We go out with whoever was there, have a good cry, and feel better in time.

LOOKING AFTER FRIENDS
- R - R - R -

"Nursing family and friends is always more emotionally taxing than nursing strangers," says Kimberly in Nova Scotia. "Any nurse will attest to that."

Lois was my good friend — we had worked many shifts in emerg together. One day her husband and daughter were side-swiped by an oncoming city bus at an intersection.

The ambulance brought their daughter, Katlyn, a beautiful seven-year-old, in before her father. She had broken her neck and had major internal bleeding, but her exterior was intact. We couldn't give up on her because all of us knew the family, but we knew it was a lost cause.

Lois' husband was brought in with a head injury, two broken legs, and a fractured pelvis. He was conscious but in bad shape. What was so difficult was the fact that he kept asking about his little girl. Lois hadn't arrived yet — she wasn't on duty so they had to find her.

When Lois came in we had to tell her that her little girl was dead. She took it badly. What could any of us do? I hugged her. It was not a good time.

We stabilized her husband and transferred him to a major trauma centre, where he recuperated. The situation was unbearable, but with time, everyone is adjusting as best they can.

WHAT'S WRONG WITH THIS PICTURE
- ℞ - ℞ - ℞ -

Lydia has been nursing in northern Manitoba for several years and is coping with the enormous challenges she faces on a regular basis. Some plights are far more contentious than others. This is one of them.

Nine-year-old Billy pulled the trigger of a .22 calibre shotgun, shooting and killing a twelve-year-old boy. We're not sure if this was an accident or if there was intent, but Billy had a history of assault.

Our nursing intervention included trying to get Billy sent out for a psychiatric assessment. The Mental Health Act dictates that a magistrate sign the required documents, but we didn't have a magistrate. And the doctor didn't feel it was necessary yet.

As nurses, we were convinced Billy needed help because he had been involved in two prior violent incidents. Two years ago, he beat up a three-year-old in a fight over "the sniff," a type of solvent.

A three-year-old kid tried to grab the sniff from a little girl and punched her. Billy intervened, demanding that he say he was sorry. When the kid refused, Billy took a rock and started pounding him on the head.

"Say you're sorry, say you're sorry, SAY YOU'RE SORRY!"

By then the kid couldn't say he was sorry. He was unconscious and bleeding. Billy continued to beat him until his brain was so damaged he had to be institutionalized for the rest of his life.

The other incident involved two friends who were on a snowmobile with him. Billy steered the snowmobile into a tree and jumped off at the last minute himself. One youngster had severe burns to the face because the snowmobile exploded, and the other had massive multiple injuries. They both had to be life-flighted out.

The psychologist who comes up for weekends felt this situation was way out of his league. Billy's parents weren't wild about him going for a psychiatric assessment because of the stigma attached to mental health problems. No one wants to see a psychiatrist or a psychologist because they think they'll be labelled as crazy.

So for now Billy is still living at home with his parents and receiving absolutely no treatment. Mental health is sadly neglected in the north.

RING THAT BELL
- R - R - R -

What happens when a highway statistic becomes real in the form of a permanently brain injured patient?

Margaret specializes in rehabilitation nursing in Ontario. "Primarily," she explains, "I work with those who are brain damaged as a result of motor vehicle accidents, drugs, or alcohol."

We were expecting the admission of a low level patient from a chronic facility. His name was Eric. High level indicates that the patient is usually ambulatory, has some sort of skills, control of either bowels or bladder, and the ability to feed himself. Low level indicates an inability to do any of these things.

Eric was in his late teens and had been in a car accident. Information was sketchy — he was a front seat passenger with no seat belt on, and alcohol was involved.

On his arrival by ambulance we discovered he was still unable to verbalize, one and a half years after the accident. His vacant stare suggested a lower level than we anticipated.

We showed him where the call bell was and asked him if he understood. Surprisingly, he blinked his eyes appropriately for yes and no.

He was totally dependent on others for all activities of daily living. He could move his arms, but they didn't always do what he wanted them to. His muscles were extremely weak.

He did not have the coordination to wash his face with a wash cloth, but he cooperated by lifting his arms for me to have his armpits washed, without fighting. He enjoyed his bedbaths, but when I washed his back or his behind, another nurse had to hold him over because he was quite heavy.

Eric was incontinent of bladder. I put a condom on him and attached it to a tube, which in turn was attached to a plastic leg bag that strapped onto his leg. He wore that from early morning till bedtime.

Because he had no control over his bowels we planned a bowel program designed to allow him to enjoy any activities as normally as possible. Every Monday, Wednesday and Friday, at six in the morning, we gave him a suppository which worked within two hours. This schedule avoided most accidents while he was up in his wheelchair. He always wore a diaper.

Two days after he came in I decided to shower him. He was so heavy it took another nurse and myself to push him across the hall and into the shower stall in the wheeled commode chair. He wore a neck brace because he couldn't hold his head up, but as yet there was no head rest on the commode. A third nurse had to support his head. We soaped him up and he got a great, relaxing, hot shower.

Eric was totally dependent for dressing, and again he cooperated. He knew if I had the left or right sleeve out and raised the appropriate arm for me. Thankfully, he was able to bridge, something all rehab patients are taught. He put both feet flat on the bed and raised his behind up while I quickly pulled up his pants.

He was extremely fussy about his clothing and would shake his head no or push me away if I brought something he didn't want to wear that day. Sometimes I would go through his whole closet before I could find something he would agree to wear. Eventually, to save time, the evening staff picked out his clothes for the next day.

Grooming, combing his hair, shaving — he was dependent for everything. Sometimes he was chesty sounding and I arranged to have a suction machine at his bedside. I had to use it more than once while brushing his teeth, but he was resistant to the suctioning and tried to push me away.

Eric could not eat any food. He had no swallowing reflex left and couldn't tell if he was aspirating food into his lungs. Consequently he was fed through a tube inserted into his stomach through a surgically made hole.

He refused to be fed three times a day. If I tried to hang a feed in the daytime, he would push me away or try to pull the tubing down with his flailing arms. With his consent we fed him at night.

I poured the cans of Jevity, a brownish-coloured food supplement, into a large plastic container specifically made for this purpose and hung it on an IV pole. The tube from this container connected to his stomach tube. His medications, whether liquid or crushed pills, were also given via the stomach tube, along with extra water.

At specific intervals we added a blue dye to his Jevity and checked the colour of the fluid suctioned out of his mouth to make sure he wasn't aspirating his feeds into his lungs.

Initially Eric used a manual wheelchair to get around. Two projections on either side of the chest area prevented him from falling side to side.

Transferring him in and out of bed was extremely difficult for me, because Eric was six foot two and I'm shorter than average. A large bath towel over my shoulder absorbed most of his drooling, but he sort of hung over me and half way down my back.

Two nurses had to lift him, turn him to do the mechanics to get him down into the chair, fasten his seatbelt, put the wheelchair legs and feet on, and make sure the headrest was at the right height for his head.

We were building up his sitting tolerance in the wheelchair from the beginning. However, he was forever wanting to go back to bed for an hour and then to get up again. So we'd get him up for one or two hours in the morning, put him back for an hour, and repeat the process many times in one day. Eventually we had to put a stop to this. It was a killer on our backs and by the end of the day Eric was tired and helped us even less.

In bed he was turned every two hours. He resisted this more and more as time progressed, and would grab the bars on the bed and push. He wanted to spend all his time on his back. I told him he had to turn, but he shook his head no, he didn't want to. So two of us turned him and positioned him with pillows.

He wanted the head of his bed down flat. This was not a wise and prudent choice on his part, because he couldn't feel the saliva going down the back of his throat and into his lungs. We taped signs on the wall above his bed saying that his head must be kept up.

Slowly Eric changed. He took part in many therapies from Monday through Friday. The hospital chaplain spoke to him on a regular basis. Occupational therapy helped him with his ability to dress and did a wheelchair assessment for proper seating and fit position. Physio improved his transfers and his sitting tolerance. Speech and Language rechecked his swallowing ability and confirmed that oral feedings were not an option. They also worked on communication devices and many alternatives were tried. The blinking was not always seen or interpreted properly. He was encouraged to shake his head, but he resisted this when he was tired.

He pointed a lot to indicate his needs, but we got into "duelling fingers." He would point the index finger of each hand in opposite directions at the same time. A communication board with the letters of the alphabet didn't work because there was only fifty percent consistency. We didn't know how much cognitive ability he had, or what his ability to recognize letters really was.

We tried a method whereby he would point to pre-printed codes. For instance, the code "OD" represented "open the door." However, his memory and cognitive deficits prevented this from working more than fifty percent of the time.

During this time a number of problem behaviours were recognized and identified. One was ringing the bell excessively. When I gave nursing care to any other patient in the room, Eric rang the bell. If I named all the things he might need or want, he shook his head no. He wanted my attention. He also abused the bell on his wheelchair.

We worked out a strategy for all the disciplines to use. We told him the ringing would be ignored if he had everything, and if he rang inappropriately, the bell would be taken from him for a certain time period. This approach worked well.

Another problem behaviour was that he would try to arm wrestle with anyone going by. We had to say "NO" in a firm voice to stop this.

A third behaviour identified as improper was sexual inappropriateness. The majority of therapists and nurses are female, and he would grab at our breasts. When we told him "NO" and pushed him away, he resisted. The doctor, psychiatrist, and chaplain — all male — spoke to him and the behaviour didn't occur as frequently. But it did continue until he was discharged and I'm sure it is still occurring now.

One night, after several months of intensive rehabilitation, Eric developed an aspiration pneumonia and we transferred him to an active hospital where he was put on a respirator in the intensive care unit. Eric agreed to the recommendation for a permanent tracheostomy.

When he returned to our unit he had to be suctioned frequently because of copious secretions. Any improvements in previously identified problem behaviours plummeted, and our strategies flew out the window.

Despite the emotional support and reassurance we gave him, it was nothing for him to ring fifty, seventy, or one hundred times in one eight-hour shift. He was frightened and nervous. We never did shower him again after he got the trach — we went back to bed baths.

The weeks wore on. As part of discharge planning, Eric got an electric wheelchair and fell in love with it. I'm sure he wanted to run all of us down in our tracks.

Arrangements were made for him to travel by air ambulance to a hospital near his home. This involved ground ambulances at either end of his flight.

The respirology technician and I discussed in detail specific measures required in-flight. I was concerned about his trach coming out because he coughed so forcefully, and the inflated cuff which normally held it in place would be deflated while we were airborne. I had to make doubly sure that the tapes from the outer cannula were tied securely at the back of his neck, and that the inner cannula was clamped on tightly.

With reports from each of his therapists and a video of his daily care ensconced in a huge bag of equipment, I left with Eric and the ground ambulance attendants on the appointed day. He required constant care. He coughed. He sputtered. His face turned blood-red.

In the airplane I found myself facing an attendant, a mere twelve inches between our knees. I jammed my portable suction machine and equipment bag within reach.

Eric was to my left. His head was two feet ahead of me.

"Do your seatbelt up, please," I heard. If I had to suction Eric, I couldn't reach his mouth with my seatbelt done up. I informed the attendant.

"Keep your seatbelt on at all times," he persisted.

Shortly after takeoff Eric started choking, flailing his arms and legs about uncontrollably, practically falling off the stretcher. Briskly, I unfastened my seatbelt and suctioned him. The attendant also unclamped his seatbelt, so he could support Eric's shoulders for me.

All things considered, Eric tolerated the flight relatively well. The ground ambulance met us on schedule, and the next time he had to be suctioned was in his room.

When I left Eric was ringing the bell.

Nurse, Hear You, Hear Me

GRIEF THAT CANNOT SPEAK
- ℞ - ℞ - ℞ -

Nurse Sandra has dedicated her professional nursing career in Alberta to looking after babies in the nursery. "It's always heart-wrenching when parents cry," she says, "but this experience was more difficult than usual."

An anacephalic baby was born, a firstborn son. The infant's head was completely open on top — no skull had formed. What little there was of the brain was exposed to the air. The doctors could offer no hope to the horror of it all.

These infants usually die within a short time because the spinal cord and the brain become infected, or the brain stem, where the respiratory centre is situated, is affected and respirations cease.

The broken-hearted parents wept and wept. As the days progressed the devastated mother said a tearful goodbye to her son and terminated her visits.

The father continued to come in daily wearing a fresh suit, shirt and tie. His shoes were polished to a high shine. My mind made an unwanted analogy with a story I had recently read — Joseph Conrad's *Heart of Darkness* — in which the chief accountant was impeccably dressed to the point of having a starched collar and cuffs. However, this form of dress was out of step with the chaos and darkness of the situation. Nonetheless, because the accountant kept up his appearance despite the circumstances, another character said he "respected the fellow."

That's how I felt about this father — I respected him. He had no control over his son's life but he gave him his personal best.

The infant died on the fourteenth day. I could not console the parents. I could not console myself.

GOING HOME
– R – R – R –

Despite every possible explanation, nurse Holly in Manitoba could not impress upon her patient the seriousness of her condition. The sick woman only wanted to go home.

Jody came to our nursing station at five in the morning as an overdose, several months following a kidney transplant. She was twenty-nine and the community health representative told me that Jody had been beaten by her husband for years. When her kidneys failed, he refused to let her go for dialysis. He didn't trust her, he said. She was placed on the kidney list.

Now, after yet another fight with her husband, Jody swallowed too many deadly pills, causing her blood pressure to drop dangerously low. Although she was fiercely combative, we started an IV, washed her stomach out, and gave her the black activated charcoal to absorb any pills still in her stomach. Protocol.

After enduring our treatment Jody wanted to go home. She said she did not intend to kill herself, she was just upset with her husband.

When we catheterized her she had next to nothing in her bladder. The transplanted kidney had failed due to the drastic drop in blood pressure and she had no kidney function left.

A nurse arrived to escort her on the emergency life-flight to the city. Jody argued. "I don't want you to send me out. I want to go home."

We did fly her out, but in the evening Jody went to her final resting place. She was free. This was the only way, her family told me afterward, that she would ever escape her abusive husband.

THE THOUGHT OF SUICIDE
- ℞ - ℞ - ℞ -

Nurse Bernice explains her professional nursing role in the Northwest Territories. "There were many stabbings and attempted suicides. My job was to bring them to the hospital for treatment."

Rarely did a doctor accompany me, but this call had such ominous overtones that I asked him to come along this time. On Christmas Eve we flew into a native settlement.

A fellow named Notaku had shot himself through the chin. The gunshot didn't kill him but most of his face was gone. Because of the seriousness of his condition we flew on to northern Alberta, where specialized medical help was more readily available than in our hospital in the NWT.

I'll never forget Notaku's eyes. He hardly had any face left except for these deep, searching brown eyes. He remained conscious and stared at me throughout.

He kept gagging on blood, but since most of his tongue was gone I could hardly tell where to suction. There was nowhere to put the oxygen mask. I aimed the oxygen flow in the general direction of his face.

The plastic surgeons worked on him for weeks and weeks, removing ribs and performing reconstructive surgery on his jaw.

Notaku survived long enough to commit suicide. This time, he took an overdose.

AN ACRID SMELL
- ℞ - ℞ - ℞ -

That's what greeted nurse Nancy in her Alberta hospital when she returned the pager after being on call all night.

My mistake was returning the pager. Once there, I couldn't leave. The nursing station was deserted.

"What's going on?" I asked a passing clerk.

"Something down in emerg," she said.

I guess curiosity killed the cat — I hurried to emerg. Waiting area full of people. Couldn't see any staff. Not a good sign. Overpowering smell. The smell of burning flesh.

The first nurse I saw was Sharon. "I need you. Get in here." Eyes hanging out of her head.

Four men caught in a flash fire, an explosion. Walked in despite serious injuries. Treatment room one, one of the men burned so badly he puffed up. Name of Robert.

First thing I saw was his eyes. Wide open. Completely conscious. Just his belt and a charred piece of pants dangling from the belt. Everything else burned off. Put a gown on and started working. Tried to get IVs started, but hands and arms too burned. Put them in his feet. Stressful.

Didn't know Robert. Sharon did. When he came he said, "Sharon, am I ever glad to see you." She didn't recognize him.

Covered him in saline-soaked dressings. Burned smell in my nose.

Had to split his fingers. Too swollen. Like cutting a carcass. Could develop compartment syndrome. Fluid everywhere. A first for me. Probably for him too.

He talked, thankful we were there. Calming effect, this talk. Pain. Gave Morphine to kill the pain.

Keep airway patent. Wife in to visit before we tube him. Stress. Talk. Tube him. Airway okay.

Waiting room full of crying. Screaming. Families. Horrible.

In our minds, it took an eternity in slow motion to get him and the other three stabilized enough to transfer to a burn centre, but they were here less than an hour before they were flown out by helicopter, and became survivors.

The smell lingers.

MOST DISASTROUS CHANCES
- R - R - R -

Jean-Paul describes an evening of "most disastrous chances" in his Quebec emergency department, an evening forever destined to remain in the annals of Canadian outrage, horror, and sadness.

One of the worst evenings we ever had in Emergency was when Marc Lepine shot some of the students at the Ecole Polytechnic. That was how many years ago?

Two of them came here. One died. One survived.

But what was tremendously difficult was initially the families didn't know where their daughters were brought, and they were coming to the emergency room to find out — "Is she here? Is she okay? Where is she?"

We didn't know. Eventually we found out from Urgence Sante, the ambulance dispatching system, but even they didn't know at first in the confusion. It was hard to know who was where.

The evening was busy to start with and to get that on top of it made it a difficult and emotionally draining shift. All the pain and the emotions of the people in the waiting room were terrible, because the news was already out.

There was nothing formal done to deal with the situation for the nurses. Some debriefing was carried out because we talked about it for the following week. It happened on a Wednesday evening I think.

It was far more than getting a gunshot wound. We get them all too often unfortunately, but it was the way it happened, how these people were attacked and murdered. Everyone was feeling at risk, especially in an emergency room open to the public where, regardless of the security we might have, someone can come in with a gun and start to shoot.

Initially people were focusing on what happened and how it happened. Later, we realized it could happen here. It's not that we wanted extra security, but we realized how one's life can be changed in a second by someone who is crazy.

What made the whole thing worse is the fact that he shot women. In a job like in the emergency, eighty-five percent of the nurses are female, with only a few male nurses. This makes it particularly hard to take.

ACCIDENTALLY
- ℞ - ℞ - ℞ -

Betty is a nurse in Nova Scotia. "I've had lots of near drownings," she says, "and a patient with a fishhook stuck in his eye. Another got his foot tangled in a lobster buoy and barely escaped with his life.

"But the shift that stands out in my mind is this one."

While driving in for afternoons in emergency I heard the wailing of fire sirens. Once at work I was told two DOAs had been brought in. There had been a head-on collision in which two cars became totally enmeshed.

One of the drivers was thrown between the two cars before he burned to death. I was experienced and had no desire to see him, but one of the younger nurses was curious. She asked me to accompany her.

His left leg was twisted around facing the wrong way, and he was wearing the charred remnants of a Mickey Mouse T-shirt. He looked like a burned roast. We couldn't get rid of the smell of burned flesh. Maybe it was in our minds, I don't know, but it was ghastly. Right now, if I close my eyes, I can still see and smell him.

The man in the second car was in his forties, and his wife and two kids came in asking to see him. Another inexperienced nurse started to take them down to the morgue.

I realized the family had been notified that he had been seriously injured in a car accident, but they didn't know he was dead. They thought they were going to the intensive care unit, not to the morgue. I caught them just in time.

THE BARE FACTS
- ℞ - ℞ - ℞ -

Grizzly bears don't attack, black bears do. That's cardinal rule number one. The exception to this rule resulted in tragedy in Alberta. Nurse Doreen relates the facts.

Hiking and camping created the perfect visit for a young British couple, until a brown grizzly bear barged out of the bush into their camp. He ignored their suppertime provisions and tore after the petrified woman who scaled a western hemlock for safety. In hot pursuit the grizzly clambered after her and, swiping the air with his five curved claws, skillfully scalped her. It was like peeling the lid off a tin can.

For his trouble of trying to rescue his girlfriend, the man was brutally mutilated. The grizzly broke cardinal rule number two — never eat humans. When the wardens got there, the grizzly was munching on the dead man's body. The left leg was missing.

On arrival in emergency, the shocked, hairless woman required sedation and psychological support. We started IV lines, cleansed her wounds, and made the necessary arrangements to transfer her to the city hospital. After extensive skin grafting and reconstructive plastic surgery, she returned home, a camper no longer.

They brought the man's body into emerg. Actually they bring lots of bodies in. People have mountain climbing accidents and fall into rivers and canyons. A lot of transients come through in the summertime — there's the occasional suicide, someone who decides to spend his last weekend in the mountains and does himself in either by overdose or by gunfire. A friend of mine was hiking and discovered a body hanging from a sitka spruce. Nobody knew anything about him — he wasn't a local.

The morgue can be quiet or busy. Last summer we had a lot of water accidents. A large canyon close to town beckons tourists without telephoto lenses. They saunter past the railings, slip, and OOPS, down they go, searching for the perfect picture. They have multiple trauma or they're dead. If they're in the water for a long time, they die of exposure.

Crevasse accidents occur in the Columbia Icefields despite "AT YOUR OWN RISK" signs. One young hiker fell into a crevasse between fifty and a hundred feet deep. By the time we were notified and sent help, the climbers found him pulseless and breathless. He was a full code, and we worked on him for hours. His core temperature was too low and he had to be pronounced dead. Losing the young ones is always hard. I had nightmares for weeks.

Unlike big city hospitals with chaplains, we provide all the psychosocial care. Ninety-nine percent of the time, we have people from out-of-town or out-of-country, and they don't know anyone. We support them while they make calls informing relatives and friends that their wife or their son has died. We become their family.

A high percentage of our car accidents are the result of people who have been driving all night for an illness or a funeral, and there's a fatality en route because someone fell asleep at the wheel.

This is all bad news, but these are the bare facts.

HELP
– R – R – R –

Does dealing with tragedy take its toll on professional nurses like Elizabeth in Saskatchewan?

"Sensations like hearing the crunching sound of a broken bone remain rooted in my memory," she explains. "Sights and smells I'd rather forget stay with me. People have no idea."

Cries for help preceded the distraught young man who ran through our emergency doors on the stroke of midnight. "Come help me. They're in the van."

People often get panicky for no reason, but this had the dark feel of the real thing. The doctor and I followed him to a black van precariously parked in the ambulance entrance.

He and his buddy were at the lake, he said, about an hour from here, and they witnessed an accident. Frantically, they threw the two victims into their van and drove here like mad.

In the back we could see a blood-drenched teenager whose head angled abnormally. We knew his neck was broken. He wasn't breathing. In the front, the buddy was restraining an hysterically sobbing girl.

I called the trauma team, grabbing a stretcher en route. The whole team came out and we rolled him in, CPR in progress.

Simultaneously we cleared his airway, stabilized his neck with a Philadelphia collar, hooked him up to the cardiac monitor, started two large bore IVs, and looked for the source of bleeding.

The monitor showed a straight line. His pupils were fixed and dilated. We knew he was dead, but we couldn't let a teenager go without a fight. We followed the ACLS protocol. I charted the time of death.

The bell at the registration desk rang. It was the boy's parents. They were taken to the front office, knowing only that their son had been involved in a serious car accident.

While the doctor talked to them I discontinued the monitor, tied off the IVs, and tried to make the boy look less sick than he was, which was ridiculous considering he was dead.

The mother fainted before she could identify her son. The father, speechless, clutched the bed rail with one white-knuckled hand, while the other gently stroked his son's dead face.

They were hit head-on by a drunk driver and didn't have a chance. The girlfriend was okay. Physically.

NEGLECTED
- ℞ - ℞ - ℞ -

"This is not a happy story, but I was deeply affected by it," says nurse Lynne in New Brunswick. "I don't think there's ever been a nurse who hasn't become discouraged with the system we're supposed to be part of. Especially where kids are concerned."

I work in emergency so I don't have long-term contact with people. We never know what happens to our patients and one of our big questions is always, "What ever happened to so-and-so?"

Jason was brought in with terrible second and third degree burns to his upper legs and buttocks. He had taken a candle to go to the bathroom because the electricity had been discontinued in their trailer. The candle was too short and caught on fire.

Jason was eight years old but he looked around four. He was filthy dirty and neglected in appearance. What struck me was that he did not cry. He didn't whimper or make any sound at all. That he was neglected was obvious. This was the cornerstone.

We're out in the country, so after our primary care, we sent him out to a burn unit for admission. After two days, however, he was discharged to the same environment he came from.

We were given the care of his burn dressings on an outpatient basis. No matter what I did to him, no matter how much I had to pick, and debride, and clean his burns, he never cried. He lay there with a resigned, withdrawn, introverted, dead look in his eyes, and let us do whatever was necessary.

He must have had a remarkable constitution because in two months, his graft site and burns healed. It took that long to get him to say "hello." I don't think he knew how to carry on a conversation. He didn't talk to his parents either. At school, he was kept in grade one for three years instead of being put into a special class.

Since then, I've probably seen him twenty times, with various injuries. Every time we report the situation to the social workers, but he's still living at home. It was so frustrating because his parents were already in the system and on social assistance.

I don't say they actively abuse their children, but they haven't got a clue, and they are untrainable. As far as I could see, Jason was left to rot. That's the only word. It seemed like social work and everyone had given up.

We've all had to deal with this type of situation, where we feel like we're beating our heads against a brick wall. I feel so angry and frustrated, I sometimes wonder why I bother. Why do I keep on doing this, day after day, month after month, and year after year?

WHAT I REMEMBER I CAN'T REPEAT
- R - R - R -

"I can't talk about the more disturbing experiences I've had on pediatrics," says nurse Rosslyn from the Yukon. "It's too upsetting."

For some reason, there are lots of children with chromosome disorders here. They often present with a low mentality and seizure disorders. Most have little brain activity, and all are difficult feeders.

They're usually diagnosed shortly after birth, either because of seizures or because they're "FLKs," funny-looking kids — this is a term I need to remember to forget.

Years ago, if they got through infancy it was a miracle, but now we have children fourteen and fifteen years old. Parents care for them and bring them back for respite care for a week or a month.

They require total care. They aren't able to feed or dress themselves or do any of their own activities of daily living. Many have gastrostomy tubes into their stomachs for feeding, although some do eat normally.

The children aren't allowed to die. CPR was done on a three-month-old boy with a chromosome disorder, while he convulsed for hours. He was transferred down south on a chartered flight. Although the child survived, his mother cannot care for him.

Today this eight-year-old is blind and deaf, has little brain activity, and is institutionalized. In these cases, what do we do, as nurses and doctors? We can't give up, but what do we have left?

We had a five-year-old near drowning from down south. The girl had been submerged under ice in a swimming pool and no CPR was done until about an hour later.

In the hospital, they did their life-saving miracle bit and resuscitated her three different times when she coded. Her mother pleaded, "Please don't do this again," but they wouldn't listen. Today the child requires total care. She remains curled in a ball like a fetus. She's alive but she's not alive.

We hear about all the miracle occurrences, but nobody broadcasts anything about all the children who are living like vegetables. Nobody hears about the families who are devastated by caring for these kids. Parents rarely stay together, blaming each other for occurrences completely out of their control. They never get over it.

Nurse, Hear You, Hear Me

As medical people, we act without thinking about the far-reaching consequences — because we can't let anybody die. I have serious problems with that. Sometimes it's better to let someone die.

231

SEVEN

STRANGE BUT TRUE
- ℞ - ℞ - ℞ -

O day and night, but this is wondrous strange!
William Shakespeare, 1564-1616

Real events can be so strange as to be unbelievable. Carol, an Ontario ER nurse, relates an episode concerning a red-headed twenty-year-old psychiatric patient who, bewildered and perplexed by the hand life had dealt him, came in to see the doctor concerning certain delusions and hallucinations that had been plaguing him.

After completing her initial assessment Carol directed him to the quiet room to wait for the physician. However, after only a few minutes, he proceeded to the nurses' station.

"If I don't see the doctor, like RIGHT NOW," he threatened, "I'll set myself on fire."

Carol encouraged him to return to the quiet room, assuring him that he would indeed be seen by the doctor soon, and proceeded to take a wailing child into one of the ORs for stitches.

Within moments the young man re-emerged from the quiet room, struck a match, and completely engulfed his lovely red hair in flames. While nurses and physicians gasped in horror, a quick-thinking lady on the housekeeping staff grabbed a wastepaper basket and threw it over his head, extinguishing the flames.

Strange but true ...

In yet another Ontario ER, a poised, well-dressed, middle-aged lady came in complaining of a snake bite to her left hand from the previous evening. She extended her hand to Arlene, the nurse on duty, for verification.

Arlene asked if she knew what kind of a snake bit her. The lady pulled out a full length, greenish-brown snake from her purse. She coiled the dead body, with its bashed in head, round and round on the registration desk.

"I threw a rock at it," the lady explained, "and stuck it in the fridge overnight. Is it poisonous?"

Strange but true ...

Each of the following has the charm of being not only strange in an intensely curious fashion, but every one of them is true to boot.

Lillian R. Tymchuk, RN

DOUBLE TOIL AND TROUBLE
- ℞ - ℞ - ℞ -

The calamitous events of one rainy summer night, when a car was going too fast and the roads were too slippery, made nurse Isabelle think she was seeing double. She is one of 1,191 nurses in Prince Edward Island.

We had a serious motor vehicle accident brought into emergency. The driver's car had skidded on a slippery curve in the middle of a particularly heavy downpour.

While we tried to resuscitate the driver the Mounties arrived, followed by a woman with three kids in tow. We thought she was probably the wife of our patient and she confirmed our suspicions — the address she gave was local.

We couldn't save her husband despite valiant efforts. The priest came to console the grief-stricken woman and the bewildered children. Together they contacted other family members. They coped as best they could with the unforeseen tragedy.

Twenty minutes later a young woman came in, sobbing, carrying a restless infant in her arms. A terrified little boy clutched her dress.

"I was told my husband was in a bad car accident," she spluttered.

Only one car accident had come in that entire day. It dawned on me that this woman must be talking about the same man. Not wanting to believe it, I

234

discussed the situation with the doctor and my colleagues. We spoke to the Mounties.

It turned out that this man had worked somewhere in the States. He had a wife and family down there, and a wife and family up here.

This particular summer he had asked the wife from the States to follow him up here in her car. What he planned to do with the two wives, I don't know. They found out about each other after his death.

Now this is PEI, and while we do have all kinds of things, they aren't usually so obvious.

A BACCHANALIAN FEAST
- ℞ - ℞ - ℞ -

Nurse Natalie took her expertise from an Ontario ICU to the warmer climes of Australia. By using her well-developed powers of observation and problem-solving techniques, she tackled a most unusual problem in a most unusual way.

We were warned not to swim around our little island on the northern tip of Australia because of sharks. We were surrounded by the Indian Ocean to the west, and the Pacific to the east. The whitetip species of sharks abounded in both.

But the wonderful blue waters were compelling and a myriad of channels criss-crossed hundreds of islands. It was an absolute paradise. Some English nurses couldn't resist the temptation and went swimming anyway.

One day it came to my attention why there were so many sharks in the channels. The hospital had one wing devoted solely to labour and delivery and birthing.

After the deliveries, all the fresh placentas were gathered and thrown into the water. Daily, the sharks were feasting at an incredible smorgasbord. No way were they going to leave such a sumptuous repast.

I raised this issue with administration and the practice stopped shortly thereafter. Instead, the placentas were burned. The sharks must have felt snubbed because they left the area shortly thereafter, doubtless to search for equally lavish feeding grounds.

A SCIENTIFIC FACT
- ℞ - ℞ - ℞ -

Giselle, one of 9,542 nurses in Nova Scotia, is used to coping with all manner of changing circumstances. She also has reason to quibble with the witty Oscar Wilde's words, "The Doctor said that Death was but/A scientific fact:"

In ICU we had a fifty-four-year-old female who was admitted with a serious heart attack. The enzymes in her blood were sky high and she was in cardiogenic shock. We did everything possible but she was unstable — a lost cause. Her three sons insisted we transport their mother to the regional centre, about an hour and a half away.

It was snowing and blowing. Against his better judgment Dr. Callaghan, our ER physician, agreed to transfer her to appease the family whom he knew quite well. He and I left under less than optimal conditions, in the back of an ambulance with an extremely unstable patient. The three sons followed behind in their car.

It was a terrible, stressful trip. The ambulance slid from side to side on snowy country roads, as her condition worsened. Three times she arrested, and three times we resuscitated her.

She was a direct admission to the intensive care unit. The waiting cardiologist got a full report from Dr. Callaghan. Within minutes, she arrested for the fourth time.

"There's no hope for this patient," the cardiologist said. "Let's call it quits." It was over.

Dr. Callaghan and I were anxious to return because of the deteriorating weather conditions. When the sons arrived, he explained that their mother had arrested four times and that she died in ICU. Tears ran down their grief-stricken faces. He told them how sorry we felt for their loss.

No sooner were the words out of his mouth than we heard, "Dr. Callaghan, call ICU STAT — Dr. Callaghan, call ICU STAT," on the overhead paging system.

He got off the phone looking troubled. He told me that after we left ICU, the cardiologist decided to insert a temporary pacemaker, and that our patient was alive.

Irritated, Dr. Callaghan didn't know what to do. "How the hell am I supposed to tell the family?" he said.

We found the distressed family in the visitors' lounge. He told them their mother was alive. They looked at us, glassy-eyed, disbelieving. Once more, we made our way downstairs to leave. We heard another page.

"Dr. Callaghan, call ICU STAT — Dr. Callaghan, call ICU STAT."

"She died," the cardiologist told him.

Frustrated and upset, we trudged off to find the family again. Dr. Callaghan told them their mother was dead, this time for real. Their anguish was palpable.

On the way home he vowed to wait until his patients were buried for three full days before informing anyone of their death. I could hear him muttering, "Never again," repeatedly.

And the poor family. The only thing that saved us was that they respected Dr. Callaghan and had a good rapport with him. It was one of those days I wished I had never gotten out of bed.

THRENODY
- Ŗ - Ŗ - Ŗ -

The unexpected happens routinely in places like emergency and the intensive care unit, but Ontario nurse

Nurse, Hear You, Hear Me

Harriet learned that no nurse can ever predict a routine shift anywhere.

My friend Beth works on maternity, and of course nothing ever happens there. They would be shocked if they ever had an arrest. Not like in ICU, where I work. I'm always kidding her about that. At least I used to.

One Thanksgiving Monday Beth was working nights with Lettie, a well-liked full-time nurse, fifty-five and planning to retire soon. Never takes any time off. Never sick.

At 4:00 A.M. Lettie complained of a slight headache. "Go and lay down for a bit," Beth suggested.

"No," Lettie replied, "I'm okay. I have to go to the john and then I'll get a coffee. See you in a couple of minutes."

It wasn't until after a routine delivery that Beth and the rest of the staff realized Lettie hadn't returned.

They checked the nurses' lounge thinking she was lying down. She wasn't there. Okay, check the bathroom. The door was open, but they couldn't get in. It was jammed. Beth called security.

Security shoved their way in. Lettie was there, all right. She had leaned over the sink, vomited, and fell to the floor. The garbage pail had wedged itself against the door. They called an arrest, but Lettie was dead.

The next night, a young mother on the same floor arrested shortly after she delivered, and died. The following morning, all of the upper-ups were in talking to the staff, who were in total shock over the two deaths.

I don't know when the third death occurred, but I know for sure that it did, because that's how things go. At least in ICU.

MOVING DAY
- R - R - R -

Lesley, a nurse in rural British Columbia, has moved numerous times, but none of her moves was as memorable as this one.

For six months we provided palliative care to an older gentleman who was dying of cancer. He lived with his son and daughter-in-law. When he passed away, they called me.

When I got there, a large yellow moving truck was sitting in the driveway. Parked beside it was the family's little red pickup. In the house, stuffed boxes and green garbage bags crammed every room. Obviously they were in the midst of moving.

The family had obtained a permit to take the body to the funeral home in their own vehicle, but they didn't have enough help to move it out of the house.

They asked the movers to help them. They were two big burly men who seemed to take everything in their stride.

"Yeah, you need some help? Yeah, we can do that, no problem."

And with that they loaded the body into the back of the little red truck, and drove off to the funeral home, no questions asked. Maybe they thought it was part of their job.

THERE'S AN ELEPHANT IN MY THROAT
- R - R - R -

Corrie, a nurse in one of Alberta's emergency departments, was buffaloed by the discovery of an elephant.

A seven-year-old girl visiting from Switzerland was brought in with her parents. Their attempts at speaking English were heroic and accompanied by various hand movements.

"Something's in her throat," they exclaimed with much alarm.

She could breath and she could talk, but she felt something was stuck there.

"What's in your throat?" I asked.

"Lucky," she said, pointing to her chest. "This."

"How big is it?"

"Lucky," she repeated. She tapped her chest with her index finger.

I examined her chest. Slightly sunburned, except for a small irregular area on her chest.

"Lucky," she said.

We took x-rays of her chest and abdomen. There, sitting for all to see, was an elephant, its turned-up trunk promising good luck for the owner.

With much gesticulation she said she got sunburned at a pool while wearing her lucky elephant pendant on a chain. When she slid down a waterslide, she fell off, breaking the chain. She swallowed a lot of water, plus her lucky elephant. Closer examination of the small white spot on her chest revealed the shape of an elephant.

There was no obstruction. She was stable. We made arrangements for her to see a specialist, and instructed her not to eat or drink anything.

We try to accommodate tourists by referring them to a centre that is close to their original destination. Her parents drove off with their lucky little girl in their rented car.

LADY BUG, LADY BUG
- R - R - R -

In computer lingo, a bug is a mistake in a computer program. Noreen, a nurse in Ontario, thought her patient made a mistake when he told her about his bugs, but they weren't in the computer.

Terry was a patient on the rehabilitation floor for spinal cord injuries. Still in his early twenties, he was an alcoholic and a drug abuser who had been pushed off a cliff. He was a high quad — his injury occurred high up on his spinal cord. The residual damage included loss of use of his arms and legs and everything in between.

A recent grad, I had been working on the floor for less than a year. One evening I spent a frustrating half hour on the computer trying to enter the patient census. The computer refused to accept what I thought was my valid password.

"Leave it for now," one of the other nurses told me. "There must be some bugs in the computer."

I found the situation strange, because the day before I sent a message to the maintenance department to repair a broken air conditioner, and the computer accepted my password with no problem then.

A few minutes later I heard boisterous screaming and yelling. Terry had been rowdy all evening and was causing lots of trouble with the visitors.

I wondered what Terry was up to now, and walked down to his room. He was screaming at the top of his lungs, "Get 'em OFFA me, get 'em OFFA me."

"Get what off you? What are you doing now?" I asked.

"Get 'em OFFA me," he bellowed. "I'm covered in BUGS." He was close to being hysterical.

I couldn't see anything. The thought crossed my mind that his troublesome friends must have given him some street drugs or possibly alcohol. It wouldn't have been the first time. He continued screaming, "Get 'em OFFA me, get 'em OFFA me."

I rolled back his bed covers. His bony body was completely covered in brown, heavy-bodied, elongated bugs. June bugs. Because Terry was paralyzed from the neck down, he couldn't shake them off. Someone must have pulled his covers up, knowing full well that he couldn't remove them without help. A small snicker sneaked out before I could stop it.

Who had closed the blinds I don't know, but they were closed when I came into the room. Upon opening them, I could see that the maintenance man had removed the air conditioner and taken it for repair. The screen was gone.

Outside, a stately Lombardy poplar was almost entirely defoliated by these pests. The window was open still and the light must have attracted the June bugs.

MOOSE IN HER HAIR
- R - R - R -

There are countless reasons for being late for work, but the one used by Alberta nurse Amy was original enough to beg future use.

In the spring and fall, our abundant wildlife create multiple problems. The fall is the rutting season for elk and the bulls become tremendously aggressive. A colossal bull with an enormous rack is frightening and I was late for work when one blocked the entranceway to the hospital. Someone inside the hospital realized I was there, and did a holler and a yell, which eventually worked.

In the last couple of years we've had more problems because the elk are more militant, bringing their young into town, and letting us know who's boss.

One of the two hospital entrances is at the emergency department. Our patients sometimes have had to wait outside because of elk obstructing the doorway.

The animals have charged at children, causing injuries. The park wardens go to the school grounds before the kids arrive and hang hockey sticks and other paraphernalia from themselves to make it look like a bull's rack. They hoot and holler and shake these racks to get the elk off the playground.

Tourists come into town looking for the park, but the wild animals are free to roam throughout town. Tourists mistakenly think the animals are tame, and try to get a picture of the kids or granny or feeding the animal. "Come on Johnny, stand close to the elk and we'll get your picture," and similar comments resulted in a seven-year-old boy being brought in, bleeding profusely. The elk gave him one good swift kick to the head, and he required forty stitches. He was lucky, he lived.

This summer, some elk set up their territory in the campground, where one readily trampled a visitor. She was not a happy camper.

It's easy to hit a moose at night because they come on the highway with no warning. In one such collision, the moose landed on the hood of the car and piled through the windshield with such tremendous force that the driver had moose in her hair. Surprisingly, she survived. The moose was dead, but often it's the other way around.

Many moose, elk, and deer are killed on our two major highways. The coyotes usually run fast enough to escape. The trains run right through town, and the enginemen say that because the trains are so big, they often don't even feel the impact. They kill a lot of bear and elk but there doesn't seem to be any immediate solution to this long-standing problem.

THE PORI-PORI MAN
- R - R - R -

Nurse Karen was in Australia for the tranquility that only the southern climes can provide, far from the pressures of nursing in Ontario. She discovered that it was possible to get too much of a good thing.

I was fortunate enough to be hired by the Queensland government, under bond. They looked after the Canadian nurses very well, and picked us up at the airport.

Aside from the large cities, much of Australia is untainted, untouched, and beautiful. The sisters' quarters were right beside the hospital. We received our accommodations, three meals a day, total laundry including uniforms, and maid service for a minimal cost.

One day Matron called me and she said, "Sister, it's time for you to go on night shift."

I hate nights. I thought I'll be darned if I'm going to work night shift for six straight weeks, with only one weekend off. Most nurses who came from the big ranches outside the city lived in the sisters' quarters and worked and slept and ate. That's all they did, and I wasn't about to do that. I went to see the liaison and told her I'd like to go somewhere else, on contract.

"Absolutely," she said. "Would you rather go to the islands or the outback?"

In two days, I was off to Thursday Island in the Torres Straight Islands, in the northern part of Australia. This was an island three miles long and populated by several thousand people. There was a handful of Caucasians — nurses, school teachers, police on rotation from the mainland, and three doctors.

No TV, no radio, and no newspapers — it was wonderful. The little wooden hospital was on the tip of the island and visible from the sisters' quarters. Matron's house was nearby.

Matron was an elderly Scottish nurse. Every morning she would start her day by sitting on her porch, her legs up, and three of the native nurses in attendance. One would be polishing her shoes, another would be doing her hair, and the third would bring her tea and the hospital report book from the previous two shifts.

Lillian R. Tymchuk, RN

That's how she reviewed the events and activities of her hospital, overlooking the incredibly beautiful blue sea, and hundreds and hundreds of islands in the Torres chain.

One morning, Matron arrived at the hospital early. "Sister," she said to me, "come immediately." I wondered what I had done now.

Because of the salt air, the wind, and the sea, one wall of the hospital had completely caved in. The view was spectacular enough to have been in the movies. Sheets were blowing in the breeze, tattered by the salt air, and the few remaining curtains wrapped themselves around lonesome window frames. In the middle of this picturesque scene was a poor bedraggled man. Sleeping. In one of the beds.

Matron said, "Sister, is this how you attend to your patients?" There was an edge to her voice.

"Matron," I said vehemently, "I've never seen this man before in my life."

Matron thought he was a patient who wasn't receiving proper care. But he was a vagrant who had wandered in, so I got a reprieve on that one.

Another day, the white police drove up to the front of the hospital. "Sister," they said, "come out to the car. We've got a real treat for you." I knew this would be good.

There is a difference between the Thursday Island natives and the Australian aboriginals. The aboriginals have a Neanderthal appearance with the broad nose, broad bridge, and slanting forehead. The

248

Thursday Islanders have a Solomon Island extraction, and they truly are a beautiful-looking people.

By his appearance, the man inside the car was obviously a Thursday Islander. I stuck my head through the window and was overcome by the smell of rotting flesh. I knew we had a big problem. The police watched me turn green.

This native had fallen into a campfire. He was so stoned on local drugs and alcohol that he was unaware of the fire. According to native witnesses, he was on top of hot coals for several hours. I couldn't imagine such a thing, but they insisted that he didn't bother getting out of the fire because he was so anesthetized.

He was perfectly conscious now and his expansive smile revealed pearly white teeth. His shirt had melded into his skin, and his skin was rotted into his shirt, and I couldn't determine where one stopped and the other started.

I asked him how long he had been like that. Four days, he said. His burns were grossly infected and almost gangrenous.

I called the native nurses to help me. They took one look and backed away.

"Please help," I said, "he can't walk by himself."

"No, Sister. We won't."

"Why not?"

"He's the pori-pori man."

Pori-pori man means witch doctor. These people were superstitious and believed in curses, bone-pointing, finger-pointing, black death, and black magic.

This man, they told me, was a well-known witch doctor from the north end of the island. If local native nurses inflicted any pain on him or displeased him in any way, they or their families would be cursed. They were firm in their convictions and steadfastly refused to help. Not one native ever touched him. White nurses provided all his pre-operative and post-operative care. That is how life is there.

Because we were so remote we relied on ourselves for entertainment. We were fortunate in that the Australian Navy came in, and the first place they showed up was at the sisters' quarters.

Those Australian officers with their blond hair and dazzling blue eyes treated us very well. They took us out in boats and took us camping. We were glad to have them there, because we all had such a good time. Nonetheless, by the end of the fourth month, I was starting to feel some deprivation — culturally, I suppose.

The patients never wanted to stay inside and were always down at the beach. As usual, I kicked off my sandals one day, and walked down to the beach to tell them to come for their medications. They looked at me like I was from outer space.

"Sister, don't bother me. I'm fishing." I yielded and brought their medications to them.

Just then a small speed boat came tearing across the channel at unbelievable speed. It swerved to a full stop, ramming the beach. Someone was in big trouble. A man and woman emerged. As I got closer, I could see the man's hand was dangling by a few shreds of skin.

We hastily phoned the pilot who was on the island to fly this man to the city for reconstructive surgery. I packed my things and took a whole valise of Demerol. There was no counting of drugs.

I loaded my patient up with Demerol, but he sat up and talked to me for the entire flight, seemingly unconcerned. He was a fisherman.

It was late at night by the time we arrived, so we decided to stay over and fly out the next morning. I was accommodated in the sisters' quarters, where I luxuriated in a lovely hot tub and comfortable bed.

Early the next morning I walked around the city, feeling like an alien. On my little island, I had been culturally deprived and without stimulation. The store windows mesmerized me. Inside a grocery store, the canned corn and canned peas got to me, and I knew it was time to leave. I was wiped out, burned out, or else I had jungle fever.

I left Thursday Island after an incredible four-month stay, and I wouldn't have traded a moment of it.

YOU TAKE THE HIGH ROAD
- ♩ - ♩ - ♩ -

Agreement on serious issues is more complex than the lines from this song suggest. Nurse Alicia's dramatic narrative from Manitoba vividly demonstrates the perplexities that can arise in trying to reach a consensus.

A plane with a pilot and five passengers crashed nine miles from our nursing station, close to the station across the lake. Although it was spring, ice covered the lake, but it was too thin for the plane to land on. The nurses there radioed over and told us what was happening.

I had four stretchers and three nurses available, but getting there was the big problem. Fortunately there was a plane on our airstrip, a relic from another time, called a "Found." The pilot agreed to fly us.

Four of the patients were already at the nursing station with a variety of injuries. We used a noisy, rattling Bombardier that easily ran over ice and snow to bring in the remaining two. By this time there were several planes around because they had called for search and rescue. We decided the best plan was to "scoop and run" with our patients.

There was a twin-engine Otter on the runway, the only one I have ever seen with carpet on the floor. We removed the seats, and four stretchers fit in perfectly. I squeezed in for the flight.

Really, I was trying to make sure the patients were all alive. I went from one to the other, doing their vital signs. When we spoke with southern Manitoba via two-way radio, it was difficult to communicate because the signals were so bad.

I knew the pilot who had crashed. We had flown together many times, transporting seriously ill patients on medi-vacs.

"Could you ask them to fly higher?" this pilot-cum-patient asked feebly. He felt more comfortable when we were higher because of the difference in pressure.

A few minutes later one of my other patients said, "I feel better when we fly low. Would you ask the pilot?"

It was up and down like a yo-yo to the cockpit. After what seemed an eternity, we landed. As soon as the plane doors opened, television cameras and the media surrounded us. It was awful.

True to form, one of my patients went flat — my pilot friend. I poured IV fluids into him and he picked up by the time we got to the hospital in the ambulance.

When I checked several days later to see how they made out, I was pleased to know that recovery was not far away.

PROTECTED
– ℞ – ℞ – ℞ –

"There's more violence in our society," states Ontario college nurse Joyce. "We're seeing that reflected in the college situation and it's indicative of the type of student we're getting now."

We recently had a situation where a disturbed patient blamed the doctor for not curing him. A mature student with serious psychological problems, he threatened the doctor and the entire health clinic staff.

"If I'm going to do anything to myself, I'm going to take other people with me," he warned.

He talked about doing something in the front lobby and it was taken seriously enough that we were being guarded.

Being guarded was what made it so funny. Our commissionaires were retired and varied in age from sixty-five to eighty-something. Only one, Dick, was in his forties. Taking turns placidly sitting in the waiting area, in plain clothes, none of them could have been mistaken for the intrepid Hercule Poirot.

Dick was like a petulant schoolchild. He didn't want this assignment and he let it be known. He sat for two hours, looking miserable, grumpy, and bored.

"If this guy comes in," he asked me, "what would you like me to do?"

A few hours later, he said, "So what does this guy look like anyway?"

After a while, we couldn't even find him. Someone thought he had gone for a smoke. The situation was pathetic and hysterical at the same time. Typically, we laughed to release the tension.

Similar circumstances are occurring in every college and university throughout Ontario, where the students themselves can be frightening.

CATHETERIZATION CALAMITY
- R - R - R -

In a hospital in the Northwest Territories, nurse Heather was taking the last step in a certain nursing procedure, only to find her patient had taken his final step.

We were short-staffed in emergency. Besides a nurse from pediatrics that I was orienting, there was the supervisor and the doctor on call.

As usual, at supper time, the medi-vacs arrived on scheduled flights from the northern communities. We assessed everybody, and concluded that in the group of five, the elderly Inuit gentleman was the most stable and could wait in ER. That way, I could give him more attention. The others were processed and admitted.

This man had never been out of his home community and had never been on an airplane. In his whole life, he had only been to the nursing station three times. Understandably, he was anxious.

He was dehydrated and his symptoms suggested a gastrointestinal flu. We decided to give him intravenous fluids, and the doctor ordered a foley catheter to be inserted into his bladder to drain his urine. Accurate intake and output could be maintained this way.

His EKG was normal, but I followed my inner feeling and put him on the cardiac monitor. After an injection to control his vomiting, he settled down and looked better.

He spoke no English, so his daughter interpreted my explanations while I inserted the catheter. Suddenly she stopped in mid-sentence. I looked up. He had arrested. In the smallest room in the department, of course. I yelled for the supervisor.

"Code Blue! Code Blue!"

The code ran picture perfect. The ideal patient, he followed the textbook and we successfully resuscitated him, but he didn't regain consciousness. His daughter was beside herself.

The poor man got sent out to a centre in Alberta, which was totally alien to him. And every time they did something invasive, he coded. Four times in all.

Periodically we heard about him — he was still in a coma. Eventually, no further news came, but we didn't forget about him.

Months later, on Christmas Eve, we got a phone call from Alberta telling us that this man woke up. They thought he was totally nuts, that something was wrong with his brain. By then, of course, his daughter had returned home, and they forgot he couldn't speak English. As soon as they got someone who spoke Inuktuk, they realized he made perfect sense.

They kept him another two months and discharged him. His final diagnosis was, "Extreme Vagal Response due to Foley Catheterization." What a ribbing I got. As a result of that incident, there are still people who refuse to allow me to catheterize elderly gentlemen.

A HELL OF A TIME
- R - R - R -

"Usually near-death experiences are positive," says critical care nurse Tiffany in New Brunswick. "This one was anything but."

After a cardiac arrest, several of my patients have said, "I felt I was whooshing through a long, dark tunnel when I saw this bright light ..." and what they see afterward gives them comfort and removes all fear of dying. But Lawrence had a different story.

Lawrence was a man who had been drinking all his life and never gave any thought to God or religion. If the truth be known, he never cared much for anything other than himself, his business, and his money.

In his early fifties, he was admitted to our facility with a heart attack, and we subsequently had to transfer him to a larger hospital. En route, his condition rapidly deteriorated and he arrested. We defibrillated him three times before he came around.

Later, he told me he remembered hurtling at incredible speed through a tunnel lined with beautiful flowers. Then he stopped — BANG.

He could hear people harling and crying, and he saw a colossal hole from which they were jumping, trying to escape. It was pitch black. Then BANG. He was back.

He didn't mention writhing snakes or flames licking at his heels, but it was enough to make him a changed man. He went to church and showed a genuine concern for others. He has since died, but before he did, he was able to say, "I'm ready now. I know I won't go to hell."

TOO YOUNG
- R - R - R -

"I've been a pediatric office nurse in Ontario for the last twenty-five years," explains Minnie, "so I've seen many little ones come and go, and grow into big ones. We have quite a group of characters that come into our office."

The mother of one of our teenage patients was overbearing, over-protective, and neurotic. She fought with the teachers every time they opened the school windows for fresh air, petrified her daughter might catch cold. She didn't allow her to go swimming in the middle of winter for the same reason.

The girl was nice, a bit timid, but we built a up a good rapport because she came in regularly for allergy shots.

One day, I could sense a lot of internal conflict going on, even though she didn't say much. I asked her if there was something she wanted to talk about.

"I want to have a baby," she said, looking at the floor.

Health teaching is important in a pediatric office. I've seen so many young girls ruin their lives because they felt the way out of a bad situation was to have a baby.

I told her that at age sixteen, the last thing in the world she'd want to do would be to get pregnant. She looked dumbfounded. I followed up with my standard lecture on birth control, but she wasn't receptive.

"Getting up in the middle of the night with a crying child is a big responsibility," I said. "Get yourself an education, then you can do whatever you want. Travel to any of the wonderful places in the world."

"No," she said abruptly. "I'm too young to travel."

COCK SURE OF HIMSELF
- R - R - R -

Jed, a hardy eighty-year-old gentleman from British Columbia, told his bizarre story on the radio, according to nurse Charlene.

Jed lived about half an hour out of town, on the other side of the bridge. He was driving his trusty truck across the bridge, swerved to avoid a bump, and hit a beaver. When he got out to see if it was okay, it attacked him.

The beaver bit him right in the crotch, tearing the artery on the inside of his right leg. It kept jumping and biting, grabbing chunks of tissue.

Thinking the beaver would bite his hands if he reached down, he grabbed a wrench from inside the truck and hit it. Somehow he managed to drive into town.

One of his relatives lived near the clinic, so he pulled in to her place. She saw him drive up, but when he didn't get out of his vehicle right away, she walked over — he's quite a character and usually bouncy. By then, he had pulled himself around to the front of his truck.

"I got attacked by a beaver," he told her.

"Jumped off a nickel, did it Jed?"

But he looked pale and his pants were torn and drenched in red. She rushed him to the clinic where I was on duty. On arrival, his blood pressure was dangerously low because of the large volume of blood he lost.

A hardy gentleman with a good attitude, was Jed. He improved rapidly and did well on the home care program.

VOODOO
– R – R – R –

In return for her nursing expertise in immunization and feeding programs, Ontario nurse Miriam deposited many unique experiences into her memory bank. Plus interest.

A group was going to Haiti for six weeks to do island-wide immunization, and I signed up. The drivers there drove jeeps across rickety old bridges made of rotting wood, occasionally making us get out and walk across. Or we'd be hurtling down dangerous mountain roads at breakneck speed in minivans, dubious brakes billowing out black smoke.

We went into the mountains and set up our clinics on church porches, under palm trees, in somebody's front yard, in a school, in a prison, wherever we could.

Our Haitian helpers advertised the immunization program, shouting to the locals in Creole through a megaphone. They provided an effective sales pitch by inviting them to bring their children and reviewing all the diseases that immunizations prevent.

Droves of people, hundreds really, started coming out of the mountains. They brought their children, who were absolute pictures out of Hollywood — scrubbed clean, bows in their hair, and wearing starched little dresses.

They did not know how to form lines or how to take their turn. We enlisted the help of the local chiefs, one of whom actually beat them off with a stick. After that, their learning curve seemed to go up speedily. They also realized that once they had their needles, they should go home and not stay around to be entertained by this local happening.

There were hundreds of people pushing. It was so bad I couldn't even lift my arm to give another needle because they were crushing in on me. At one point it was so hot, and I was so sweaty, I thought I had literally lost it. I had to break through the hordes to collect myself.

Many beautiful Haitian children lived in orphanages. We had a feeding program in one centre and gave each child a bun and a sliced banana. That's all these kids had to eat for the whole day.

One thing that struck me was the setup of the graveyards. Many of the grave sites had cement houses with steep, sloping roofs. They said it was to keep the dead in, to prevent them from being the walking dead — zombies. The whole issue of voodoo and zombiism is prevalent in their culture and they have a firm belief in it.

After people have been buried, they later have been seen walking across fields, or around villages where they were born. This is inexplicable.

In Haitian folklore, a zombie is a soulless corpse who can be reanimated by a Voodoo priest, and then does his bidding. While many discount these stories, others say that a powerful poison, a neurotoxin which comes from the puffer fish, is used to paralyze the victim into a deathlike state by stopping all vital signs. In powder form, it is easily absorbed into the body through the skin or through ingestion. However, when analyzed, this powder has very little or no poison at all in it.

Supposedly, one of the initial reasons for zombiism has to do with slave labour. People were given this drug, buried, and somehow resurrected shortly after. Of course, their brains were completely fried because of the drug and probably from lack of oxygen, and then they could be used as slave labour in the sugar cane fields. Apparently zombiism has its beginnings in this type of story.

"SAONIQ"
– R – R – R –

In Quebec, nurse Francie came to the shocking realization that her little patient was said to be an incarnation of her — but Francie was still very much alive.

In the village, I have my *saoniq* which literally means "it's your bones." An Inuit woman who was close to me adopted a little girl and named her after me. It is an honour for me to have my *saoniq*, and incurs no specific responsibility.

When little Francie wore her first hat, her mother gave it to me. I like to wear bright colours, and her parents dress her in similar colours, and keep telling her that she's me. It's something else.

This is a difficult concept which can only be compared to reincarnation — except that I'm still alive. Little Francie is said to actually be me, and because I'm a nurse, she's considered to be a nurse. When she was a few weeks old, the elders would say to her, "I have a cold. What should I do? Will you take care of me?"

This belief went so far that I had to interfere. Two men about my age were touching the little girl on her chest when she was two years old, while making believe it was my chest.

"Leave her alone. If you want to touch me, you come to me. I'm the big girl. She's not me." I knew they would not touch me, but when they saw her, they saw me.

One night little Francie's mother called me in the middle of the night. "I'm jealous," she said, "you're sitting on my husband's lap."

"What are you talking about?" I demanded angrily. Then I realized she was talking about my *saoniq*. I wondered what would be called incest in a situation like this.

I learned a lot — it opened my eyes. Before we use the word incest, we have to see what it means for a particular culture. There used to be a lot of incest here, with the elderly touching the infants, and I wonder if it was because of this concept.

That was the traditional way with the old generation, but it's changed with the new one. Now they're all mixed up with our culture and our religions.

ALREADY DEAD

— ℞ — ℞ — ℞ —

On Prince Edward Island, nurse Nicole deals daily with a variety of patients in the outpatients department. Mildred is one of them.

Mildred was a tired-looking, forty-nine-year-old who wore cotton floral housedresses and carried a large brown vinyl bag, regardless of the season. She constantly pushed straggly hair from her line of vision. At home, she cared for an elderly father.

At outpatients, she usually presented as fairly functional, but she had numerous physical complaints which had been investigated repeatedly. It got to the point where none of the doctors on call wanted to see her.

"Mildred is here."

"I don't want to see her. There's nothing wrong with her. We've investigated her and its costing a fortune." But they would see her and eventually send her on her way.

Mildred refused to see a psychiatrist, and because she wasn't a danger to herself or others, we couldn't admit her or have her certified.

One day, when she made yet another visit to out- patients, one of the more experienced GPs was on call and he agreed to see her.

"What's wrong with you today, Mildred?" he asked her.

She looked him straight in the eye. "I'm dead, doctor."

"Well Mildred, I guess if you're dead, dear, there's not much I can do for you, so you might as well go home."

Content, she returned to her home.

Lillian R. Tymchuk, RN

HIS, HERS, AND I'M NOT SURE
- R - R - R -

"One of the things I love most about working in the college setting is the infinite variety of students," reflects Ontario nurse Debbie. *"Not to mention the bizarre happenings."*

A female student rushed into the clinic one morning anxiously jumping from one leg to the other and bending her knees at the same time.

"Can I use the washroom in here? Please?"

In a few moments a more composed student re-emerged. "Can I talk to you?" she asked.

She went on to express a great deal of concern about using the women's washroom outside one of the classrooms. She said she had gone into one of the stalls when she noticed a pair of pretty pink sneakers in the next stall that were headed in the wrong direction. The person obviously was facing forward to urinate. She bolted out of the washroom without completing her task and ran to the clinic.

The person she described was well known to us, a tall, heavy-boned student who had changed from being Phil to Phyllis. Phil now dressed as a female, sometimes in jeans, but more often in a long flowery skirt topped by a soft-looking blouse or a delicate sweater. His/her blond hair was longer now and gently curling up at the ends, and he/she liked to wear a little bit of red lipstick, some black mascara, and just a touch of blush. It was more difficult to exactly pinpoint his/her perfume but it smelled expensive.

To date, he/she hadn't had any corrective surgery, just hormone therapy. However, his/her lumberjack's gait and deep voice did nothing to enhance his/her feminine side and consequently Phyllis looked and sounded like a great big man in woman's clothing. He/she caused a lot of anxiety around here.

I would expect a person who is in the transitional stages of changing from being he to she, but who hasn't had the surgery yet, to continue using the male washroom but I guess it would be difficult to enter wearing a skirt. There are no easy answers. Maybe we need three washrooms.

CAN YOU HELP ME
- ℞ - ℞ - ℞ -

When a nurse burns out because of constant stresses and lack of professional support, a special patient sometimes comes along to make her realize she is in the right profession. The patient who turned things around for Alberta nurse Diane wasn't able to communicate with her. Was he?

It's easy to get cold and callous in a neurological critical care unit, and I knew that was happening to me. Things just didn't affect me as much anymore.

Peter was my new patient, a twenty-two-year-old with Down's syndrome. He was running across the street to catch a bus when he got hit by a car. He came in with a severe brain injury and had to be ventilated. He was not doing well.

In caring for Peter and interacting with his parents and brothers and sister, I felt so much love. He touched many lives with his special gift in his short time. A myriad of friends and acquaintances showed great strength.

Someone from the family was with Peter day and night, and they appreciated every little thing that was done for him. I looked after him every shift I was on, for ten days, until he died.

He somehow got to me and although I can't explain how or why, he reaffirmed the reason I was in nursing and why I had chosen the neurosciences field, as tragic as it can be.

We'd had a terrible year with patients dying traumatic deaths, and I found most of the staff had shut themselves off from emotion.

Peter and his family made me care again, although he never regained consciousness. I interacted with him only as nurse does with a comatosed patient, but in talking with his family and friends, I could sense so much loving and caring that I was amazed.

My husband realized something important was going down at work because I got quiet at home. Not quiet-withdrawn, but quiet-thinking about things.

After Peter's death I felt rejuvenated in a strange way. I knew I had supported his family and friends during a difficult period, but I also knew the extent to which they encouraged me. This experience gratified me and kept me in nursing.

SEE ME, SEE YOU
- R - R - R -

After the following experience in British Columbia, nurse Roberta pondered whether or not we each have control over certain events in our lives, and whether we attract specific situations to satisfy deep-seated inner needs.

Recently, my fifty-five-year-old patient Sylvia lost her sight. Her husband had retired a couple of years ago, but had done nothing to prepare himself for retirement.

He was thwarting the care we were giving her. At the conscious level, he didn't realize what he was doing and I don't believe he did it maliciously. But he needed her to be blind, to look after her, to give him something to do to keep the house going.

I don't think people realize what they're doing sometimes. They behave in seemingly rational ways, but when you examine them closely, serious questions arise.

Previously, when her two older sons were leaving home, Sylvia became pregnant again. She was emotionally detached from her husband and needed someone else in her life. The only thing she could think of was screwing up on her contraceptives and having another child. When I confronted her with that, she agreed.

In her blindness, she complained about the way her husband guided her. It was obvious how uncomfortable she was with him, but she wouldn't say anything to him. She feared hurting his ego to the extent that he might start drinking again.

She asked me to intervene, but I said no. She had her own reasons for acting the way she did — as did he — and they continued on as before.

EIGHT

SUPERNATURAL GOINGS-ON
- ℞ - ℞ - ℞ -

And Nurse came in with tea-things
Breast high 'mid the stands and chairs —
But Nurse was alone with her own little soul,
And the things were alone with theirs.

Sir John Betjeman, 1906-

In a profession so strongly linked with life and death
nurses provide priceless support to their patients,
especially when given a healthy nudge by the unseen.

The supernatural makes its presence known
through the senses of unsuspecting nurses and patients.
The sense of sight causes the chosen to stare in disbelief,
to rub their eyes and perhaps subconsciously try to make
an uneasy vision go away. The sense of hearing can trick
the selected ones into saying, "I must be hearing things."
Right answer, wrong interpretation.

Strong unexplained feelings may present as a
sudden awareness of having to do something or to be

somewhere. Feelings of apprehension, received in either the sleeping or waking states, may forebode impending tragedy.

The inexplicable results of the unseen are often left for nurses to contend with, without explanation. To make life easier nurses lump together premonitions, strong feelings, dreams, and even belief systems under "intuition." There are fewer questions this way but nurses who act on their intuition can intervene in beneficial ways on behalf of their patients.

When the past brushes up against the present the results are as electrifying as thunder and lightning. Numerous nurses confront supernatural beings during dark and eerie night shifts, and consequently they have definite views on the subject. "Of course I believe in ghosts. I've seen too much not to," is a typical observation.

Michele, a nurse in Alberta, argues that there is an abundance of evidence to substantiate such a belief. "Our hospital is on the main floor," she explains. "The cafeteria and the maintenance department are way down in the basement.

"Every time I work nights, between 4:00 and 5:30 A.M. the elevator comes up to the main floor from the basement. The door opens with a squeak and a crank, pauses long enough for someone to walk out then surreptitiously makes its way back down.

"Other times I've gone to the basement to get a bite to eat and the microwave would be on and running. No food is ever in the microwave but the light is on and the mechanical 'Huummmm' is on with about three minutes left to go. No one else has been down there."

In each of the true stories that follow, nurses share a variety of baffling incidents that occurred while they were carrying out their professional duties.

HEAVENLY HUE
– R – R – R –

Was the room blue? Were the flowers really there? If they were, where did they come from? Did Mary, one of 24,268 nurses in Alberta, actually see them? These puzzling questions remain unanswered to this day.

Cathy, a lovely nine-year-old girl, was diagnosed with cancer and subsequently had extensive chemotherapy. She was much loved by all the staff.

For many months she was in extreme pain and her beautiful face gradually changed, becoming haggard and wan. Her dying dragged out for many weeks. She came from a strong religious background and had a Catholic family who was very attentive to her.

Cathy died on the evening shift. The charge nurse said, "I've washed Cathy up. Come now if you want to see her."

I had trained in a children's hospital and had seen many other children die. I wasn't afraid and we were all fairly well prepared for her death. But as I stood in the doorway I was totally overwhelmed by an awesome feeling.

The room was not painted blue but it was blue that day. The strong blue ambiance brought forth a spiritual connotation. And there were bouquets of flowers and garlands that I didn't recall seeing before. I was mystified. Where had they come from?

Cathy looked peaceful. Children often look beautiful when they're dead, unlike some elderly people. In my undecided agnostic heart I felt this little girl was okay, that she was going somewhere nice. Everything was all right with her and she was going to have a great time.

In retrospect I don't know if the flowers were there or not but the other-worldly sensation of that room has never left me.

Since then, in my reading, I've learned that blue is one of the colours in the spectrum that is peaceful and spiritual.

GHOST NURSE
- R - R - R -

The following account was related by Sharon, a nurse who is always cool and poised in the most stressful of situations. She works in a large, old hospital in Ontario which used to house tuberculosis patients and was later changed into an active general hospital before its final demise as a chronic facility.

"I've come across numerous unexplained events as have most nurses who have worked here for a while," she muses, *"but this was the strangest episode of all."*

When I was working in the intensive care unit we cared for a critically ill patient by the name of Bill, who was in his late forties. He had suffered a serious heart attack. We weren't sure whether he would survive but we thought he might talk himself to death if he didn't take a breather. He talked non-stop.

One night he was talking aloud although his room was empty. He hadn't received any sedation recently.

"Who are you talking to, Bill?" I asked. "There's no one in here. Try and get some sleep."

"I was talking to the nurse standing at the foot of my bed."

"None of us were in your room, Bill. Go back to sleep."

Thankfully his cardiac monitor showed normal sinus rhythm. I adjusted his bed covers, covered him with an extra blanket for the night, made sure his bedsides were up, and joined the other nurse at the nurses' station outside his room.

The next thing we knew he was standing at the side of the bed. Surprisingly his cardiac monitor had not alarmed with his movements, and although we hadn't heard any noise, one of his bedsides was down.

He said he wanted to go after the nurse who was just in and ask her some more questions. He explained that for the last couple of nights he had been talking with his deceased father and that this nurse had stood at the foot of the bed. She had said to him, "No, you won't be going to see your father. It's not your time now. You'll be all right."

We helped Bill back into bed and after that night he didn't see or talk to anyone else. He ultimately recovered.

We never heard any more about the ghost nurse. A number of times, however, I've heard footsteps, especially on nights, and I would think that either a supervisor or security was coming, but no one ever showed up.

Several nurses have seen little flits of white. Once when I was coming out of the intensive care unit on my way down to emergency, I saw a little bit of white going around the corner, like a uniform or a lab coat. No one was there.

THE PREMONITION
- R - R - R -

Premonitions involve knowledge of future events. Someone may have an idea something is going to happen but is unable to give a rational explanation.

They may present as strong feelings which can work for the benefit of patients as Sally, a busy ICU nurse in the Yukon, found out.

To this day I cannot explain the premonition I had about one of my patients. We only have one surgeon up here. When we're busy, he's busy. At this particular time he hardly got any sleep because of the number of critical patients in ICU.

On the night shift I was looking after a patient who had abdominal surgery following a gunshot wound and he was progressing relatively well. His vital signs were stable. He seemed fine but I felt something was not quite right and expressed my concerns to the supervisor.

"Keep an eye on him," she advised.

Half an hour later, I called the surgeon.

"I really have nothing specific to tell you about this patient but I feel there's something wrong," I said, half expecting an angry blast in my ear.

However, the surgeon came in and we ended up taking the patient back to the OR and putting him on a ventilator. For days it was touch and go but eventually he was discharged, a healthy man.

The surgeon claims I saved this patient's life because I listened to my feelings. "Don't ever worry," he said. "If you feel funny about one of your patients, that's good enough for me."

GOODBYE
- R - R - R -

Every mortal doesn't complete his work before moving on. Diane, a nurse on a spinal cord rehabilitation centre in Ontario, describes one such occurrence.

Jim and I developed that special connection that comes with working together for fifteen years. He was an orderly. We could say anything to each other and know that it would be understood and accepted.

My husband didn't like him but he didn't have to worry. Jim was gay. Five years ago he was diagnosed with AIDS.

Until Jim needed help, I didn't know when he felt sick because he never told me. When he was admitted to the hospital he rhymed off certain people that he didn't want to come and visit him and I was one of them.

That was okay. One of his closest friends called me and said, "It's only because he doesn't want you to see him like this."

I saw Jim only once in the last few months before his death. The last time we spoke, he didn't say goodbye. The funeral was a private affair.

Three days after he was buried I was on afternoons. A bell went off in one of the empty rooms while we were making rounds. I turned it off. The bell went on again. I knew there was nobody there so I returned to the desk and turned it off again.

Once more the bell went on. This time I knew it was Jim. I entered the room feeling chilled, light-headed, and a bit weird.

"Come on, get out!" I yelled. "No more nonsense!"

The bell never went on again. I knew it was Jim so I didn't feel particularly scared. I think he did this to say goodbye.

LITTLE GIRL
– R – R – R –

Shelley is a pediatric nurse in Manitoba who finds something positive about every shift. The following experience however, left her in a state of astonishment.

My friend Ruth and I often did our nights together and we welcomed each other's company and expertise. This night was no different.

All of the children were sleeping peacefully. The IVs dripped soundlessly with each passing minute. Everything was under control.

The play room was pitch black since all the lights had been turned off hours ago. I was walking though it to join Ruth at the nurses' station when out of nowhere, the illuminated form of a little girl appeared beside the toy box. She looked my way momentarily and without warning, faded from view.

Heart pounding against my rib cage I returned to the nurses' station, afraid to turn around yet wanting another look.

"What's wrong with you?" Ruth asked. "You look like you saw a ghost."

"I did. I mean — I saw a little girl in the play room and then she disappeared right before my eyes," I whispered.

"What did she look like?" Ruth demanded. She was in charge now. I explained that I saw was a beautiful little girl about five years old, with blond curly hair.

Ruth rifled through her purse and extracted a crumpled picture. "Is this who you saw?"

I was dumbfounded. "How did you know?"

Calmly Ruth explained that the little girl — Ashley — had been a cancer patient there before I came. She used to love playing beside the toy box with Ruth and the two had developed an unwavering attachment to each other. Ashley had died one year earlier, to the day.

ALWAYS SAY THANK YOU
- ₿ - ₿ - ₿ -

Cheryl is an orthopedic nurse in Ontario who knows everything about broken bones and how they heal. She is well aware of the infinite ways her patients can say thank you to her for providing excellent nursing care — sometimes they thank her verbally, occasionally present her with a box of luscious chocolates, and sometimes even bestow her with an affectionate hug.

However, one of Cheryl's patients thanked her in a way that she had never heard of before and never wants to encounter again.

Mrs. Notta was a delightful lady with a fractured hip on the orthopedic floor where I worked. She wasn't doing well post-operatively because of pneumonia and other serious complications.

I had completed my evenings and was getting ready for seven gruelling nights. During that time our rotation was seven evenings, seven days, seven evenings, seven nights. Over and over again.

Mrs. Notta had no family of her own and I spent as much extra time with her as possible. We developed a strong bond that was rewarding for both of us.

After two busy days off I returned on nights. My special patient wasn't mentioned on report.

"What happened to Mrs. Notta?" I asked.

"She died on your days off," the evening nurse told me.

At the time I felt not a sadness but more of a relief for Mrs. Notta because she had been in pain. She was an elderly woman who had lived a full life.

I went ahead with my usual duties, and at five o'clock in the morning it was time to get the ice waters organized so I could whip them around before doing the required vital signs — temperature, pulse, respirations, and blood pressure.

Everything was dark. The lengthy hall was pitch black all the way down to the murky sunroom, illuminated only by a flickering red neon EXIT sign.

As I crossed the corridor between the nurses' station and the kitchen, I glanced down the dark hall ... and I saw Mrs. Notta!

At least I saw half of her. She was filmy down below but I could plainly see that it was her. There was no colour to her. She was pale — ashen really — but I could easily make her out.

I sucked my breath in, in total shock. As I stared she smiled and waved to me. It was the biggest smile, like she was at peace. Then she literally floated into one of the end rooms and that was the end of it.

I didn't wave. I didn't do anything. I stood there, stunned. I thought afterward maybe I should have waved but at the time I was numb.

Needless to say I was shattered for the rest of the shift. I grasped the kitchen counter with sweaty palms, trembling, panting. What did I see? I rubbed my eyes. Was it the night shift? Was I going out of my mind?

I told myself to settle down — right now. I made two executive decisions: I wasn't going to walk down that hall, and I wasn't going to breathe a word about this to anyone.

Near the end of the shift the patients' lights started going on with the usual requests, but I made myself scarce and the other nurse had to answer them all. I couldn't go.

I think I was in such shock that I didn't know what I was seeing. If I started reflecting, I knew it was Mrs. Notta. It was her face. Previously, certain peculiar places had evoked a feeling of apprehension in me but never had I seen an apparition.

The situation wasn't threatening in any real sense and she never returned. Later when I had a chance for calm deliberation in the safety of my own home, I felt she must have been telling me, "It's okay. I'm going on. Thank you."

POLTERGEIST IN THE O.R.
- ℞ - ℞ - ℞ -

"The first part of the bowel surgery — a sub-total colectomy — went fine," says OR nurse Cecilia in Alberta, *"but soon the poltergeist was harassing this surgeon again."*

I scrubbed meticulously with pink stanhexadine for a full five minutes. The first case of the day was a seventy-year-old woman with a malignant tumour. Inside the OR the circulating nurse already had the surgeon's favourite Mozart tapes playing — Symphony No. 40 in G Minor, to be followed by Symphony No. 41 in C Major — "Jupiter."

After donning sterile gown and gloves I arranged all my sterile instruments first on the prep set, then on the front tray and back pan that were placed on the Gerhardt table which slides over the OR table. We did our first count of the day — ten small reytex, ten larger reytex, bovie tip, three blades, Metzenbaum scissors, curved and straight Mayo scissors, one reel.

Then the instrument count — three sponge sticks, ten kellys, eight kochers, three allis, ten mosquitoes, six lowers, Coolly forceps, long finger forceps. Retractors — Harrington, right angle, Jackson. Bookwalter. Five babcoks. Needle drivers — three long, two medium, two short, and so on.

As soon as the patient was anaesthetized we put in an art line, a CVP line, and a catheter. The residents helped position, drape, and prep her. We started.

"Scalpel." Incised the skin, with a #20 blade.

"Bovie." Cauterizing tissues and vessels while delving into the abdomen. The surgeon talked about his family's recent trip to Boston and how his kids liked the whales.

"Two kochers." Down to the peritoneum.

"Harrington retractor."

"Right angle retractor." Deeper and deeper into the abdomen.

"Bookwalter." Attached the retractors to its ring circle; nobody had to hold them now.

"St. Mark's Retractor." Large retractor with six inch blade. Used deep down in the bowel toward the sigmoid colon, in the supra-pubic area, to lift up and get good visualization.

"St. Mark's Retractor!" Wrapped separately, kept in one particular spot only. The circulating nurse can't find it. Running between rooms, searching. It's not there.

"Get me the ST. MARK'S RETRACTOR!!"

I know it's the mischievous poltergeist again. Doesn't like this surgeon and always play pranks on him. Surgeon is now antsy, becoming nasty. I smile behind my mask.

"Is it too much to ask for the headlight or can't you find that either??" Snarls. The bright headlight goes on.

More bleeding than desired.

"Cooley forceps!" No teeth. Used for holding fragile tissue.

"Bovie!"

Transfused two units of warmed blood that was run through the warmer.

"Kelly!"

"Kelly!"

"Scissors!"

"Tie!"

Located the tumour, cut the bowel with a stapler system called a TLC-75.

"Reload!" Four lines of tiny staples very close together. Specimen out. Irrigated the abdominal cavity with warm saline.

"Pool sucker." Two-piece suction system that sucks up water and doesn't damage delicate tissues. Start to close.

"Number one Vicryl." Closing instrument count. Skin count of sponges and sutures. Dressing in place. Patient is wheeled to the recovery room. Mozart is turned off.

An hour and a half later the St. Mark's retractor is found on a cart where nobody would ever, ever put this instrument.

My belief in poltergeists is substantiated by my reading. I always think the Maritimers have quite a bit of fun and games because poltergeists are quite prolific in the United Kingdom and there's the theory of "hands across the water ..."

MARY
- R - R - R -

Do Maritimers have fun and games? Patricia is a pediatric nurse in New Brunswick who will most certainly attest to Cecilia's suggestion.

Patricia found when she was short-staffed that help from the ethereal in the form of the ghostly Mary was better than being on duty by herself.

Around the turn of the nineteenth century the old hospital in New Brunswick had long narrow windows and huge open wards. There the school of nursing turned out new nursing graduates every year.

Mary, a student nurse in those early days, was working on the pediatrics wing which was situated on the eighth floor. She had several infants in her care and like all student nurses, felt the overwhelming pressure of her workload. She had babies to feed and babies to change. And how they were crying.

To get her assignment done Mary picked up a bottle and put it into the mouth of the tiniest baby, propping the bottle against the pillow. Then she did the same thing for another baby, who a minute before had been crying his little eyes out. She knew that propping babies like this with their bottles was absolutely forbidden.

The results were disastrous. The tiniest babe in her care choked to death. When poor Mary realized what had happened she threw herself out of the eighth floor window and killed herself.

Ever since that night Mary has returned in spectral form and has been looking after the infants to make sure nothing like that has ever happened again. There probably hasn't been anybody since — myself included — who worked in that nursery who hasn't had some type of encounter with Mary.

One night while I was charting, the charge nurse was checking a new admission. Suddenly one of the emergency call bells rang out. I rushed to find one of the babies choking. He was already cyanotic. I cleared the baby's airway just in time to avert sure disaster.

I wondered who could have sounded the alarm. One of the infants? The charge nurse at the other end of the floor? Right.

Students usually got the assignment of working nights in the nursery along with one grad. If ever a student started to doze off, she would literally feel someone shaking her by the shoulders — when nobody was around. This happened all the time, whether or not one of the babies was in trouble. Mary again.

I saw the empty rocking chair in the nursery start to rock as though someone sat in it. People who didn't work nights said it was the wind. People who did work nights knew it was Mary.

I could feel her presence in other ways. Coming out of the formula room I would often feel the swish of her long full aproned skirt going by.

One night during supper in the cafeteria I had an overpowering sense of urgency to return to the floor. I paid heed to my feelings and discovered one of the babies had spiked a high fever. I was able to provide the proper nursing care before the baby became more ill.

We weren't ever supposed to prop babies like Mary, did but it happened. One of my friends was assigned to four screaming babies. She tried to prop one up but no matter what she did, she couldn't get the bottle into his mouth. An unseen someone kept taking the bottle out.

That part of the hospital has now been abandoned and a new regional hospital has since been built. I don't know what happened to Mary but she certainly has provided part of the folklore of that institution.

TINK-TINK
- R - R - R -

Ghosts have been known to return to once familiar haunts when renovations are taking place, as evidenced by Laura's account from Ontario. Her methodical and analytical approach is one Sherlock Holmes might envy.

I used to do a lot of nights on the medical ward that had reopened after extensive renovations with Beverly, an RNA.

At half past one in the morning one of the older gentlemen got out of bed to go to the bathroom and knocked his hand on a bedside table, causing some paper-thin skin to be torn from the back of his hand. As per protocol, we were obliged to report this incident to the night supervisor who responded immediately to our call.

The patient was duly seen to and put back to bed. He was quite sane and compus mentus. The supervisor said, "I'll come back later for the incident form. I have a few other stops to make."

At precisely five minutes past 3:00 A.M. — I had just documented the time on the incident form — Beverly and I heard footsteps coming down the corridor from the top of the ward. Neither of us said anything since we were expecting the night supervisor to return.

The footsteps became louder with a distinct "tink- tink-tink" noise, stopped momentarily in front of the nursing station, and disappeared round the corner.

Neither of us clued in that we hadn't actually seen anyone. "I think that's one of the patients," I muttered. "We'd better go and check."

Flashlights in hand we checked each room. All the patients were sound asleep. We searched the lounge thinking an intruder might have entered.

Then we started to realize certain things: a) we hadn't seen anyone; b) the footsteps seemed to have come from the old type of nursing shoe that tied up in front, had a slight heel and made a "tink-tink-tink" noise with each step; c) we hadn't heard the fire doors opening at the end of the corridor.

When the supervisor returned I asked her if anybody had recently died in the hospital. She was known to be psychic and had seen a number of manifestations herself.

"No, why?"

I explained what had transpired and she said, "Footsteps often follow me around. Actually I'm quite used to it."

She believed the ghost was a former head nurse who had dedicated a lifetime to caring for her patients.

"Don't worry," she said. "She won't hurt you. She comes and has a look whenever things are being renovated or changed in any way."

Neither Beverly nor I felt any fear or apprehension. It was just one of those things.

FOCUS ON INFINITY
- ℞ - ℞ - ℞ -

Some nurses have had dying patients who seem to focus on infinity. Chrissie is one such nurse in New Brunswick. A petite blonde, she never doubts her encounters with the supernatural. She accepts the events as a matter of course in the constant cycle of life and death that she sees every day.

Just before some patients die — whether they've been conscious or unconscious — they see something at the foot of the bed and then focus in the distance. There's no doubt in my mind that they see something or someone we don't.

Eugene was dying from leukemia. His family, devout Christians, faithfully visited him every day. Sadly, his youngest daughter had died from cancer a few years previously.

When he lapsed into a deep coma I was put on to special him as a private duty nurse. He was totally unresponsive for many days despite full medical treatment.

Then the strangest thing happened. Eugene came to and called me by name. As well as being my patient he was a neighbour of mine from my home village.

"I can't believe how good I feel, Chrissie," he said.

Oh yes, here we go, I thought.

He put his deathly pale head back on the pillows and closed his eyes. Suddenly there was a glow about him and all the lines disappeared from his face. He looked perfectly serene despite the suffering he had been through.

His lips were moving but he wasn't saying anything out loud. He appeared to be having a conversation with someone he knew very well. He looked beyond the foot of the bed, then off into the distance, stretched out his hand, and died.

This experience reinforced something for me — perhaps an afterlife exists and death is merely another dimension for all of us.

STRANGE GOINGS-ON
- ℞ - ℞ - ℞ -

Shirley, a bubbly outgoing Ontario nurse, is probably about the last person anyone would ever connect to strange goings-on.

The orthopedic floor where I worked followed the L-shape commonly found in the old wings. The nurses' station was in the corner of the L, and the short leg was comprised of two private rooms that we used exclusively for confused patients. There were no washrooms there, only sinks for handwashing.

All nurses soon discovered that every confused patient ever admitted to either of these rooms used to see things none of us ever did and their stories were amazingly consistent. It was creepy.

These confused disoriented patients each said they saw a little boy beside the sink. Nobody on staff, including the older nurses, knew anything about him.

These patients also said they saw "people wrapped up" in the corner of their rooms at high ceiling height. We took this to mean bodies wrapped up in shrouds since wrapping the deceased in shrouds was part of our nursing care. That was the only way we could relate to what these patients told us.

We kept extra stretchers along the wall in the short corridor with additional supplies of sheets stacked on top. Two nurses always went together around that isolated corner on evenings and nights.

One night my friend Karen and I were working. Our orderly for that stretch of nights was Joe, a hulking six foot two university student. Karen and I were completing our 4:00 A.M. rounds by checking on a particularly confused patient. As Karen and I huddled together she was ever so slightly ahead of me.

We rounded the corner when a white form slowly took shape and rose from one of the stretchers. As I looked on in disbelief, Karen raised her flashlight high above her head and bonked the spectral form right on its scary head.

We escaped to the relative safety of the nurses' station, and who should we see but Joe, dragging a wrinkled white sheet. Knowing how frightened we were, he had played a trick on us but he paid for it with a big bump on his head.

THE WHISPERER
- ℞ - ℞ - ℞ -

Nurse Elsa derives her name from the popular Swedish and Spanish forms of Alice, which means "truthful." Elsa's story from Alberta is so unique she has no reason to be other than truthful.

I have a knack for starting IVs — older people with paper-thin skin, redheads with no veins, convulsing infants, it's all the same to me. I never miss. And my patients say they never feel any pain when I give them an injection — it doesn't matter what the medication is, even Bicillin or Gamma Globulin which usually hurt a lot. This is simply what I do best.

When I first started at the hospital I met Dr. Jones, a caring, competent, and particularly dedicated physician. He was well liked by the nurses and he never forget anyone's name.

"Good morning Dr. Jones."

"Good morning Elsa."

One morning he called me to start an IV on an infant who was bleeding profusely following a circumcision performed by an over-zealous physician. The others were unable to get a line in but I easily slipped one into the infant's tiny foot, and we replaced the fluid loss before serious problems arose. The bleeding stopped.

When I saw Dr. Jones the next day I said good morning to him as usual.

"Good morning Sister," he replied.

I asked my head nurse what that was about and she said that any nurses Dr. Jones felt a particular professional respect for, he would call "Sister," and that I should feel honoured. From that day forward he always called me Sister.

Last year Dr. Jones became terminally ill and my heart ached as I had to use my skills to start an IV on this kind and gentle man, and to give him various medications for pain control.

"Thank you Sister," he said gratefully. A short time later he died peacefully in his sleep.

A week after his death I was walking past his room and I heard someone whispering "Sister" distinctly enough that I whirled around, startled. There was no one there.

The second time it happened I was again walking past his room. It sounded like Dr. Jones and it made me feel as if I was doing everything right, that he was approving of me.

This has occurred numerous times since his death and has no particular rhyme or reason to it, in terms of what I'm doing at the time.

I mentioned it to his wife who smiled appreciatively and was very accepting of what I told her. I think it's just a different way of remembering a person.

Lillian R. Tymchuk, RN

DISEMBODIED
- R - R - R -

Voices with no apparent source make it troublesome for surgical nurses like Vivian in Saskatchewan to determine where personal safety ceases and the descent into danger begins.

Report from the evening nurses was unexceptional — here were only three fresh post-op patients. The other night nurse and I began our rounds at midnight.

In the first room all four patients were sleeping soundly, either courtesy of Mother Nature, or, more likely, from the intravenous Demerol and Gravol given by the evening nurses.

In the darkness of the hall we heard indistinct voices coming from the room occupied by one of the fresh post-op patients who was recuperating from major surgery. What we heard sounded like a macabre "he said/she said" routine.

"Mmmnnn, jbbber, jbber, ssh mn!"

"Vvrrrts wngn ravvvbn tmmrrn?"

"Mmmnn, ssh, mn, jbbbbr, jbber!!"

"This isn't a hotel," I complained to my colleague. "Why don't people leave when they're supposed to?"

Visitors were supposed to be long gone and neither of us were amused to think that someone had deliberately stayed past visiting hours. But the room was empty save our patient and she was sleeping comfortably. I consciously ignored the frigid air I felt streaming past me.

Within minutes the same indistinct ghastly voices emanated again, this time from an empty room across the hall.

"Mmmnnn, jbbber, jbber, ssh mn!"

"Vvrrrts wngn ravvvbn tmmrrn?"

"Mmmnn, ssh, mn, jbbbbr, jbber!!"

We marched in boldly with our flashlights but a sense of extreme unease began to grip us. An extensive search uncovered nothing and we were left feeling jittery and apprehensive.

At 4:00 A.M. we heard the same bone-chilling dialogue arising from the dirty utility room. This time we called security.

Together we searched each room and found no source for the voices. "Have you heard anything about ghosts around here?" I asked security.

"Don't believe in ghosts," he muttered. "That's stupid," and he hustled off the floor as fast as he could. We were no wiser — or safer — than before.

After giving report to the day staff I grabbed one of my friends and told her what had happened with the voices. She paled a bit about the mouth. "The last time I was on nights the same thing happened to me," she said. "It's been going on ever since that accident came into emerg last year when a husband and wife died. It really gives me the creeps," she said.

It's nerve-wracking to hear things when there's nothing visible going on. I had heard some vague stories about ghosts on this floor before but I never gave them any credence. I do now but I can't say that I like it.

WITCHCRAFT
- R - R - R -

This experience occurred in a huge teaching hospital in Ontario where medical entourages are an everyday occurrence — specialists of every description, senior residents, residents, interns, junior interns, medical students, and so forth.

Louise, the nurse who relates this incident, shares a sense of amazement concerning these events.

A few years ago when I worked in the intensive care unit and primary care department, I came across an inexplicable incident.

A man by the name of Brian told his family doctor he was one of a coven of witches. He claimed another witch had cast a spell on him that was making him sick.

He was manifesting real symptoms and was definitely ill. The doctor tried to treat him as an outpatient but without success. Eventually the doctor admitted him to psychiatry. After two weeks Brian became progressively worse and eventually lapsed into a coma.

We received the unconscious Brian in ICU where he became totally unresponsive, stopped breathing, and had to be put on a respirator.

No family members came but the visitors he did have professed to belong to the coven of white witches Brian belonged to.

"We're here to help," they said.

Their offer was met with skepticism by the doctors. Specialists of every type had been called in. Brian went for test after test but the doctors couldn't discover the reason for the elevation of temperature, the sweats, the rashes, the unconsciousness, and the inability to breathe on his own.

After a while the doctors finally agreed to let the witches assist, mumbling, "Well okay, if you think this stuff will help."

The bed was in the centre of the room and the white witches wanted to know the exact location from which we gave our care. With great precision they drew a symbol on the floor with a black magic marker.

They asked us to give the nursing care from either inside these markings on the floor, or if we were standing farther away from the bedside, to stand outside these markings. We were never to reach across the lines. We took care to respect their instructions.

They brought holy water and uttered incantations. Who knows what happened but Brian slowly got better, regained consciousness, and was discharged. The doctors never did come up with a diagnosis that I ever heard. Was it the witches or was it the medicine?

CONSIDER THE LILIES
- R - R - R -

Flowers brighten up the starkest of surroundings and bring bliss to the beholder. A word of warning, however, from Saskatchewan nurse Barbara.

We had just had a series of deaths on our medical floor and the emotional strain was starting to show on all of the nurses.

One day after we had passed out the lunch trays to our patients, I heard a commotion at the nurses' station.

"What are you doing? Give me THAT!" snapped one of the nurses. With that she yanked a beautiful red and white floral bouquet from the arms of a junior aide who was being oriented to our floor.

"What's wrong?" she blustered. "I was just taking these flowers to a patient."

Seeing me coming up the hall the other nurse said, "You tell her. You're supposed to be orienting her!" With that she stomped off into the utility room clutching the flowers. She re-emerged shortly afterward carrying two separate bouquets in small vases and took them to the patient.

What this aide didn't know was that nurses have always been superstitious about the red and white colour combination in flowers. We prefer to separate the red from the white flowers before taking them into a patient's room. Not to do so means another death will soon come. The other nurse obviously felt we had had enough death on our floor already without tempting fate any further.

My sister — also a nurse — died last year. Two days before her death she said to me, "If any red and white flowers come to my funeral, don't put them out. Somebody else will die and I don't want that."

THE HAUNTED HOME
- ℞ - ℞ - ℞ -

Meredith is a VON nurse in Ontario who admits to encountering weird vibes in the homes of some of her patients.

Oddly enough, I had no disturbing feelings in the apartment despite the strange events my patient disclosed to me. Jeanine lived on the fifteenth floor of a huge apartment building. While making french fries she had suffered second degree burns to her hands and required regular dressing changes.

She told me her husband had recently died in a car accident and that she had a four-year-old son. When a pot of grease caught fire, Jeanine's instant reaction was

301

to grab the flaming pot and run out to the balcony with it. She didn't want her son to get burned.

She divulged more with each dressing change and I began piecing together a bizarre story. One day she said, "I think this place is haunted."

"What makes you say that?"

"Well," she said, "look at the evidence. The french fries were on the stove and they exploded. The other day I went to pick up the kettle and the whole handle came off. All of the screws came out at the same time. Last night my gilded mirror came crashing down."

"How come?" I asked.

"I was sitting watching TV and all of a sudden this mirror comes down on me. There was strong piano wire holding it. It snapped in two. How could that happen? I know it was solid when I put it up."

She continued, dismay in her eyes. "Last week my son started screaming about the curtains. They were sticking straight out, parallel to the ceiling. No windows were open."

"Could it have been a draught?"

"No way. And there are noises, like banging on the doors, all the time."

Jeanine said she went to see the superintendent but he didn't want to talk. Friendly before, he became defensive now.

She started asking around and found out the previous occupant of her apartment had burned himself quite badly in a fire but no one seemed to know if he had survived or not.

The straw that broke the camel's back happened a couple of days later. Jeanine's neighbour said, "You had some fellow that burned himself last night, eh?"

"No. What are you talking about?"

"Well, you did," the neighbour continued, "because I saw him running out of your place, screaming that he was on fire. I went down to the lobby to see if somebody got him an ambulance but nobody was around by the time I got there."

Jeanine said that was more than she could handle. She told me she was moving and within the next week she was gone. Her burns had healed to the point where she no longer required regular dressing changes.

THE BIG ONE
- R - R - R -

Both patients and nurses can have premonitions about death. Jill, an intuitive and experienced emergency room nurse from Saskatchewan, has this to say about that.

Many times while driving in to work, if I had the idea we were going to get a Big One in, I would be right about eighty percent of the time and have an absolute night from Hell. I knew it was going to happen before I got there. I felt it in my bones.

One afternoon I had this feeling of unease while driving into work. I knew we were in for it. When I got there the usual run of injuries and medical problems demanded my attention for the first couple of hours.

And then it happened. A head-on collision involving four teenagers in one car and the driver of another. It truly was a shift from Hell. One teenager was brought in DOA, a second teen died within half an hour, and a third died shortly thereafter. The fourth miraculously escaped serious injury.

The driver of the second car was a gray-haired sixty-seven-year-old lady whose chest was impaled by the broken steering wheel column. Massive head injuries rendered her unconscious. Questions arose as to whether a heart attack had caused her to veer into the path of the oncoming car. By the end of our shift she too succumbed to her injuries. The feeling in my bones had been dead on.

But patients know things ahead of time too. No matter how trivial their concerns seem, if they look me in the eye and say, "I think I'm going to die," I know I'd better get help pretty fast because they're going to code or come pretty close.

One morning an athletic-looking thirty-year-old man came in complaining of abdominal pain. Based on her initial assessment the triage nurse had correctly triaged him as "urgent," not "emergent." As I was drawing blood and starting his IV before sending him for x-rays, his dark soulful eyes searched mine. "I'm going to die," he said. "Will you help me?"

"I promise we'll do everything we can to help you," I said. He grasped my hands gratefully. "Thank you nurse," he said.

Within minutes an undiagnosed aortic aneurysm ruptured. I kept my promise but it was not enough. He died.

It always happens without fail. Somebody, something is telling them that this is the Big One.

RECURRING NIGHTMARE
- R - R - R -

No one is exempt from having terrifying dreams which result from anxieties relating to work. In northern Manitoba, nurse Finola had disturbing dreams that she finally dispelled by confronting her distressing situation head-on.

When I first came to northern Manitoba I used to have a recurring nightmare about a woman who was admitted with false labour pains. This was before I had much experience in delivering babies.

One night we were weathered out. Hurricane-force winds prevented me from sending Connie, my pregnant patient, out to a larger facility so I kept her overnight in the observation room. I prayed that our radio and telephone lines would not go down.

I went to bed with the idea of checking Connie in an hour or so and fell into a disturbed sleep. I dreamt that when I checked my patient, I delivered her baby boy but he was like a slippery greased pig that I couldn't grab onto. Only the uncut umbilical cord kept him on the bed.

As I reached for him, he turned into a girl and then back into a boy again. I saw the new mother and her husband looking at each other, wondering what kind of a nurse I was.

With a start I woke up. It was only twenty minutes since I last checked Connie but I decided to look in on her anyway.

"Why are you bothering me?" she muttered sleepily.

"You won't understand but I've got to make sure the baby's not coming yet."

Nothing was happening and Connie had a good night's sleep. By morning the storm had subsided and she was discharged. As I gained more experience, my fears subsided and the nightmare never recurred.

THE CLOCK HAS STOPPED IN THE DARK
- ᴙ - ᴙ - ᴙ -

On Lily's palliative care unit in Ontario, patients who could not communicate with each other described a ghostly "nurse" in the same exacting detail. She appeared to have an explicit mission and it all started with the clock.

Years ago an old Ontario family lost a young girl to illness and presented a grandfather clock to the hospital in her memory. Strange things started happening when the clock was moved to our medical and palliative care unit. The ten private palliative beds are on one end of the floor and the nurses' station is in the middle.

I was working nights with Carley, a Jamaican nurse who knew something about voodoo. In the private room at the end was a soft-spoken lady named Matilda who, since her pain was well controlled, never rang her bell.

In the next private room was Father Saransson, a priest, and next to him was a young lady with cancer of the cervix. The day shift had inserted a small catheter for her that now refused to drain properly, so Carley and I were going to put a three-way catheter in and irrigate it.

As we were doing this procedure, we heard, "YE-YE-YE-YE-YE-YE," in a deep loud voice, like an exorcist.

"Who was that?" I asked.

"I don't know," Carley replied.

"Do you think it was Father Saransson?"

"I doubt it."

I went through the kitchen into his room where he was sitting on the side of the bed looking out the window.

"Are you all right?" I asked.

"Yes."

"YE-YE-YE-YE-YE-YE-YE," came the sound again.

It was more like a chant than a scream and this time I knew it came from Matilda's room.

"Matilda, what are you yelling about?"

She was looking out into the anteroom.

"I've been trying to wake up that nurse over there and she won't wake up!"

"Over where, Matilda?" I asked.

"Sitting over there on the couch."

"There's nobody there, Matilda … can I get you anything?"

Matilda was calm. To her this spirit was real. "I'd like something to help me sleep."

I met Carley coming out of another room. "What did Matilda want?"

"Tell you at the nurses' station. I'm getting her some medication and you're coming with me."

When Matilda yelled again we both ran into her room.

"What's the matter?"

"Lily, that nurse won't wake up."

"What does she look like?"

"She's tiny with short black hair."

"How do you know she's a nurse?"

"She bathed me."

"Now Matilda, you actually felt the water?"

"She washed the front of me. Not my back. But I think she's just being nosy, Lily."

"Did she speak to you?"

"She said, 'I understand you can't walk very well.' And that's true, that's what frustrates me the most."

Actually Matilda did have trouble with her legs and walking was painful.

"Matilda, here's your pill. Try to get some sleep."

"Okay Lily."

That was the last we heard from Matilda that night. Two days later she died.

Afterward I was telling one of our part-time RNAs this story, and when I described the ghostly nurse, her eyes widened.

"Describe her again," she said cautiously.

I did.

She said, "Lily, when I went in to bathe the man in the end room, he said a nurse had already bathed him. He gave the same description."

The following day he died. Oh boy, I thought, this is getting interesting. Was she cleansing the patients before they died? The story was going around and it frightened the staff. Although none of our patients were afraid, we were careful not to talk about this spirit in front of them.

Recently we admitted a lady who had secondary cancer in the bone and was taking mega doses of Prednisone. One morning she rang her bell just before report and Miriam, one of the nurses, answered it.

On her return she was visibly shaken. She said her patient told her, "Miriam, I just had a nurse come in wanting to bathe me but I told her no because it takes two nurses to bathe me and two nurses to turn me. She couldn't do it by herself."

This patient apparently wasn't ready to die and refused to be bathed. The following day an elderly lady in the next room died.

Our ghost took to asking me for help. We admitted a new patient with AIDS and sometimes they're frightened, especially at night. I was going to check on him about three in the morning. I walked past the quiet room where the grandfather clock was and I almost froze. It felt like I had walked into a fridge and right out again. I blundered on. I must have walked right through her.

"Nurse, I need some assistance in here." The voice was unfamiliar. I felt a prickly sensation on the back of my neck. Quickly I checked on my new patient and thought, it's pitch black in there. If he needs anything else, he's going to have to ring. On the way back I encountered the frigid air once more.

"Nurse, I need some assistance in here."

I didn't care what she wanted, I kept on walking. I asked my colleague if she had heard anyone talking. No, she had not.

There was only one real sighting by a staff member. Edie, a friend of mine, works permanent evenings. She was making her last rounds to make sure everyone was settled. One of the new patients had someone sitting on a chair beside her bed. Edie saw a face that seemed filmy rather than solid, but what struck her the most was the big eyes overflowing into bony eye sockets.

Edie kept on walking until she realized nobody should be in that room because the family had gone home. When she returned the chair was empty. The only way anyone could have left the room without Edie seeing them was through the window.

The next day this patient died. She had been close to death and couldn't have communicated whether or not she had been bathed.

One night I was working with a young nurse, Lee, who was frightened by all these stories. In the wee hours of the morning I answered a call bell. As I was putting a nice warm blanket on one of our older gentlemen, Lee appeared at the door.

"Lee," I said sarcastically, "I'm quite capable of doing this. I took *How To Apply Blankets 101*, you know."

"I'll help you."

She walked so close to me that I felt like I was piggy-backing her.

"What's the matter with you?" I demanded.

"Lily, when you got up from your chair, someone sat in it."

"Lee, it's a cushion chair. It must have been the air coming out of it."

"Someone sat in your chair."

I approached the chair and said, "I'm sorry, you can't sit here. You'll have to sit somewhere else."

You have to be polite to these spirits because you just don't know. I believe they are real.

Some nights the ghost set off the alarms on our IV pumps, one at a time. I would troubleshoot a pump and get it running again. The minute I returned to the desk, I heard the familiar BING! BING! of the alarm. What fun that night was.

On Thanksgiving Day Bob, a young RNA, came to relieve because we were short-staffed. He came on our floor around seven to get an early start. When I arrived he was white as a sheet, in earnest conversation with the two night nurses.

He told us he had gone into the lounge for a coffee and there was a tiny nurse with short black hair reading the newspaper. He bent down to pick up a used tea bag that had fallen to the floor, and when he straightened up, she had disappeared. There is no back door to the lounge.

"Bob," I said, "that was our ghost. She walked right through you."

He never worked on our floor again.

Our ghostly nurse is still around after four years. Maybe some day we'll find out about all this. No one will ever convince me that what the patients saw was a result of drugs and or a lack of oxygen to the brain. I've seen too much.

NINE

THE TRUE NORTH
- R - R - R -

*O tell her, Swallow, thou that knowest each
That bright and fierce and fickle is the South
And dark and true and tender is the North.*
Alfred, Lord Tennyson, 1809-1892

All Canadian nurses who work in the true north never underestimate the dark power of nature in its rawest form, but each of them exclaims over the wonder of the land and of the people.

What can we include in the true north? The provinces which reach up to or extend beyond the 60th parallel — British Columbia, Alberta, Saskatchewan, Manitoba, Quebec, and Labrador (Newfoundland).

Still farther north is the Arctic Circle, an imaginary line that runs parallel to the equator. Here, there is continuous daylight for fifty-seven consecutive days in the summer, and total darkness in the winter.

The territories are also in the true north. The Northwest Territories cover a land mass equal to one-third of Canada, extending from the 60th parallel to the north pole. A fascinating mixture of five main groups of people speak nine official languages. Luckily most understand English.

The Yukon Territory was originally a district of the NWT. The coldest temperature ever recorded in Canada was on the morning of February 3, 1947, at Snag Airport in the Yukon, a frigid minus sixty-three degrees Celsius.

How do Canadian nurses get there? By planes of one kind or another, usually. Then there's the Dempster Highway, the only North American public highway above the Arctic Circle, a frontier road of gravel, dust, and mud.

BEST FRIENDS
- ᴙ - ᴙ - ᴙ -

Nellie, one of 588 nurses in the Northwest Territories, was asked by the doctor to accompany her on a medi-vac which turned out to be the most harrowing experience of their lives.

We got a call in emergency about a woman with a rigid abdomen. She was a teacher in a community much farther north than we were. She continued to have positive pregnancy tests, even though she had a negative ultrasound before she went back up north. It sounded like a typical tubal pregnancy — an ectopic.

We do have a medi-vac service, but they were short-staffed and their two nurses were already out on call. This service is run by St. John's Ambulance and employs full-time nurses who are paid a bit less than we are because they're not unionized.

Nurses do this for the adventure and for the learning experience. Most usually stay less than five years. Having to haul heavy patients around on stretchers, at all times of the day and night, would wear anyone down. I certainly couldn't do it on a regular basis.

However, when the doctor asked me if I would accompany her in getting this woman, I agreed. We didn't think about what we were getting into. We just knew that the patient would surely die without surgery. This doctor and I were good friends. We're about the same age and had both recently married. We each called our husbands and explained that we were flying up north and we would probably be back in about twelve hours.

We flew with two young pilots in a little KingAir. The pilots said this was their best plane and the one they were most proud of. It normally seated eight, but when we pulled out all the seats from one side we knew that would leave little room for us to work in.

It was early spring and at home the weather was great, but en route billowing blizzards swirled into scary whiteout conditions. The whiteness of the snowstorms was impossible to distinguish from the whiteness of the tundra. It was frightening. Half way to our destination, the pilots said they didn't think we would be able to get in.

"We'll have to turn around and fly fuel-efficient to a different community," they informed us.

"What's fuel efficient?"

"Half the speed and twice as long." But they too were concerned about our patient.

"What's going to happen to her if we don't get her out?"

"She's probably going to die."

They decided to continue. "We'll fly up there and try to land. Once."

We tried to land five times. We would come out of the clouds, see the tops of a few houses, and pull up again. I have a strong stomach, but I was close to losing it. My doctor friend and I were clinging on to each other for dear life.

"It's a good thing our husbands are friends," she said, "because I don't think we're ever going to see them again. They can keep each other company."

It was so rough that all the alarm lights came on, and the pilots were visibly shaken. Somehow, though, we landed safely. When we climbed out we realized how close we had come to crashing — we were just two feet from the edge of the runway.

Our patient was in the nursing station in critical condition. She looked about eight months pregnant because her belly was full of blood. The nurse there had managed to get one IV line in, and I had a hard time getting a second one in because she was in shock, but I did. We gave her medication to get her blood pressure back up to normal and stabilized her as much as possible. It was imperative we not waste any time in getting her out.

The RCMP came to assist. We had so much equipment we needed extra help. We drove her to the airport in the back of a pickup truck. I sat beside her with all the IVs inside my coat to prevent them from freezing.

There was something else. The batteries on my IV pump didn't want to work in the cold. Up there it was a bitter twenty-five degrees below, while at home it was zero degrees Celsius. We weren't used to doing medi-vacs out of the hospital, and in our concern for this lady, we forget about the cold we were likely to encounter. It was a long ten-minute ride.

The snowstorm subsided and takeoff was smooth. Thankfully, so was the return flight. We were never so happy to see the hospital where we wheeled our patient right up to the OR for surgery. She did well. Neither the doctor nor I have ever gone on another medi-vac. We both felt we could do without that type of experience in our lives.

I'm from Alberta. I'm one of those who came up to the NWT quite young, planned to stay only one year, and then go back to school. I proceeded to get married and have a baby and we're still here. It's been a good place and I've certainly learned a lot because I get the opportunity to do much more than my friends down south. We're a great deal more independent here.

In June, the twenty hours of daylight are great. I don't want to go to bed at night and neither do the kids. The other night at work, it was three in the morning when we kicked some kids off the helicopter landing pad. These are nine- and ten-year-old kids who should have been home in bed.

The farther north you go, the longer the kids are allowed to stay up. They can go to sleep whenever they want. If they want to stay up, they stay up. They also go to school when they want to go to school. It's much less structured than we are used to.

The long hours of light do take some getting used to. I have to put black garbage bags on the window for my two-year-old, and he still doesn't want to go to sleep before ten. It's a fight from eight-thirty on.

In the winter, we hardly want to get out of bed because it's dark so much of the time. We don't have total darkness though. In late December, we'll probably have three hours of light, from noon till three, and the rest will be dusk or dark. The street lights on our street are usually on by three in the afternoon.

It gets me down, especially when it's bitterly cold. Last winter just about did me in. It was forty degrees below for about eight weeks, and dark. The price of power keeps us from leaving the lights on all the time. We try not to use more than we need. This winter was awful because we were plugging vehicles in all the time.

Several years ago, the choice of foods here was very limited. I remember getting excited seeing a nice sweet potato, but now we get everything. My parents were surprised that the shopping here is like down south. More expensive, but certainly as good and as fresh.

My husband isn't a hunter, but a lot of people around here fill their freezers with caribou for the winter. Good caribou is so delicious, it's out of this world. Muskox isn't bad, but it's not my favourite. Trout, pickerel, and Arctic char make sensational meals.

There's nothing like living and nursing in the north. I wouldn't trade it for anything.

"I GOT IT AGAIN"
– R – R – R –

Confidentiality is more difficult when large numbers of people are involved, according to nurse Cindy in Newfoundland/Labrador. Add to that something of a sexual nature, and your work is cut out for you.

This happened in the highest parallel I ever worked, where my patients were mainly Inuit. One morning an unknown gentleman came into my nursing station.

"I got it again," he said.

I didn't know him, but I knew what he was talking about. I knew what he had. Calmly, he told me he had been treated for sexually transmitted diseases before. My mind swirled with procedures I had to do. First was the taking of swabs from the infected sites.

Unless the plane was poised on the tarmac ready to take off to the nearest laboratory, I might as well throw the swabs in the yard because they would be useless, and it could be up to a week before a plane arrived. Nonetheless, I followed proper procedure.

With sexually transmitted diseases, it's important to contact all partners. In my best professional manner, I said, "Now Mr. Jones, if it's possible, could you name any partner you've been with since your last treatment twelve weeks ago. I will discreetly inform them that they may have been in touch with an infection, and ask them to come in for treatment. No names will be mentioned."

He proceeded to give me a list of women from one town to the next, up and down the coastline of at least seventy miles. Trying to seem worldly, I wrote down all the names.

I treated him and sent him on his way with a bag of condoms, inviting him not to have contact with anybody until his treatment was completed — and ever after.

I rushed over to Gwen, the public health nurse. "Look at this list. How are we ever going to reach them all?"

She knew the procedure for contacting the outlying areas, and I called the six women in our settlement. "I have reason to believe you've been in contact with an infection. Could I trouble you to pop down to the nurses' station and we'll chat about it?" Without using Mr. Jones' name, I got all of these women to come into my clinic.

After treating them, I discreetly asked for names of any intimate contacts. Not one of the six named Mr. Jones, but they named twelve others. With my delicate upbringing, I thought nobody would ever believe me.

But Gwen had a plan to eliminate some of them. "Otherwise," she said, "we might as well treat everyone all the way up and down the coast."

However no matter how much I begged, Gwen stubbornly refused to divulge the details of her strategy "until later." I knew she was getting a good laugh at my expense and was testing my problem-solving techniques at the same time.

I imagined receiving a call from the medical officer of Labrador — "What's going on up there? You want another case of condoms? Do you have an epidemic? You can't possibly need another four thousand capsules of the antibiotic of the day."

YING-YANG
– ℞ – ℞ – ℞ –

In Alberta, nurse Lisa is used to working closely with the RCMP, but she finds some requests more unusual than others.

Our small hospital is half an hour from the British Columbia border. An RCMP officer called from BC asking if anyone had come in complaining of pain and teeth marks in his ying-yang.

"Excuse me?"

The Mountie explained that they were searching for a man who had forced a woman to perform oral sex at gunpoint. In the midst of this violent act, she clamped down as hard as she could. But she had some sort of upper denture that came out, and the man ran off into the bitter cold with his gun and her denture, in severe distress.

"If you see anyone walking around with teeth in their dink, be sure to let me know," the Mountie requested.

WATERMELONS
- R - R - R -

"This was my initial foray into public health and community nursing, and I looked after some aspects of prevention," says nurse Gail in the Yukon. "I also looked after emergencies on the Alaska Highway."

Young and inexperienced, I had just graduated from a big city hospital in the east, but I knew I wanted to work in the north. I went to a tiny community on the Alaska Highway.

Early in spring I was called out to a highway accident fifteen miles south of my community. An unconscious man with a severe head injury paid a high price for an evening in the local beer parlour. With the help of untrained highway personnel, I transported him to the health centre in an old Dodge ambulance.

The doctor on call advised me to take him south. South meant northern Alberta. A Canadian Airlines plane, en route to Whitehorse, had already come and gone, so I had to search around for another airplane.

A newly-built mine site had a Beech 18 twin-engine aircraft that serviced the area. The pilot agreed to fly us south, some twelve hundred miles. The weather was wretched that evening, but I boarded along with the pilot, co-pilot, a mechanic, and my patient.

We followed the highway, flying at three hundred feet. I had started an intravenous, but I had no oxygen, suction, or other equipment of any kind. My teeth were chattering with the cold, and the mechanic was kind enough to loan me a pair of his greasy coveralls.

We landed in northeastern British Columbia after a very rough flight just before six in the morning. Knowing we must be starving, a good-hearted doctor there proffered greasy hamburgers for breakfast. He took one look at my unconscious patient and said, "Carry on, don't stop here. This man is not in good shape."

An ambulance was waiting for our "mercy flight" at our destination in Alberta. I was dog-tired and had been sick on the plane. At the hospital an immaculate nurse greeted us. "This is the mercy flight from the Yukon?"

I nodded. She scrutinized my grubby coveralls and the black circles under my eyes. "Who's travelling with this patient?"

"I'm the nurse escort."

"You're a nurse?" she asked incredulously.

Doubtless, my city colleagues were used to seeing nurses from mercy fights dressed in parkas. While they were professional here and competently took over the care of my patient, there was a total lack of comprehension as to what we had been through to get there.

The neurosurgeon understood. He invited me to his home for a delicious home-cooked meal that his wife prepared. They treated me like a tired daughter and offered to drive me back to the airport for the return trip.

"Is there anything you'd like to pick up before you head back?" he asked solicitously.

"We don't get much fresh produce," I said. On the way back we stopped at the local market where I picked up all my favourites — the biggest, juiciest, green and white striped watermelon I could find, luscious strawberries, and wonderfully tantalizing tomatoes, cucumbers, squash and zucchini.

We took off immediately. Although the sun was bright there was lots of turbulence. I had no way of tying my precious watermelon down, so it rolled all over the aircraft.

Fifteen minutes in the Alberta air and we were diverted to the Northwest Territories to pick up a man with a fractured hip and pelvis, the result of a caterpillar tractor accident. We flew him directly to Whitehorse and then carried on.

In a short time, we had flown from the Yukon to British Columbia, to Alberta, to the Northwest Territories, and back home to the Yukon. We were weary and exhilarated at the same time. I didn't know any better then.

INTERCULTURAL RESPONSIBILITIES
- R - R - R -

On a reservation in northern Manitoba, adventurous Nurse Trevor says, "The biggest differences between working here and in the south are the intercultural aspect and the additional responsibilities of not having a physician. Both factors took work, and I'm not sure which of the two I got used to sooner."

I honestly believe nurses in the city have no decision-making power. They have the background and the ability to do so much more. Within a year of graduating, I had reached a point where I was perishing, lost all interest, and nursing was just a job. So I went north.

Working in a different culture makes for quite a change, especially if you compare an Indian reservation to a large city like Vancouver or Toronto. Nurses here have to learn an increasing number of skills to cope with the additional responsibilities.

Here, emergency management is number one. We need to be able to stabilize patients and provide first-line emergency care, like suturing lacerations and dealing with trauma.

Officially we don't do any deliveries. We have a policy where the women are flown out to the city two weeks prior to their confinement dates. Those with babysitting problems may secretly fly themselves back with their own money, and then show up here later, in labour. To avoid this some women hide their pregnancies from us, get no pre-natal care, and come in at the last minute.

Most deliveries are routine and handle themselves. We can't stop the baby from coming out, but we can assist the mother. We stabilize the situation, make sure the baby is breathing, check the apgar score. Give the baby some vitamin K and mom some Syntocinon. As soon as the baby is delivered he gets shipped out to the city.

Compared to my city hospital experience in obstetrics, there is no difference in the quality of care. Everything is the same, but it's a completely different environment. There is a delay with regard to the physician checking everything, but the mothers are more comfortable because they're in their own community.

There's no rush-rush here with obstetricians, midwives, doctors and nurses. In our university lectures on post-partum care there was a lot of stress and commotion around new formulas, new little packages of all sorts, and vitamins.

Here, we deliver the baby without the commercial aspect. What a difference. All we want is a healthy baby, and mom to feel comfortable with what's going on.

We work as a team and have group discussions if we're not sure what the best course of action is. We follow strict guidelines, especially regarding medication. They don't just send anyone up here and say, "There you go, do as you please."

For instance, we don't prescribe chronic medications. These patients see the doctor when he visits every two weeks. It's different on each reservation — farther north, the physician visits less often, maybe only once every six weeks.

Ojibway is spoken here, and because of the language barrier, the whole interviewing process for obtaining a medical history is changed. We communicate through the CHR (Community Health Representative) or get someone else who speaks English.

Even if two-thirds of the people speak English, they do so in a concrete, operational way and find it difficult to express abstract thoughts. If we ask about quality of pain, we can't expect an answer to this type of question. Because their way of communicating doesn't translate well, we often don't get the whole story and there are many mix-ups.

For instance, one patient, escorted by a young translator, was brought in with non-specific medical problems. Typically, he didn't give me any information himself. I asked when he was born and the answer was, "in the autumn." To him that was important. He didn't know how old he was — the age he gave me was off by five years, as I discovered later from his old charts.

The following situation outlines the cultural differences and the expanded role of nursing in our setting. At five in the morning a seven-month-old baby, in his grandmother's foster care, came in as a possible overdose. While an adult relative was babysitting, one of the five-year-old kids in the house gave the baby some medicine. The bottles of Fer-in-Sol, an iron preparation, and Tylenol were found empty.

We didn't have the antidote for iron overdose that was recommended in the protocol. We pumped his stomach, irrigated it, then infused activated charcoal to absorb any lingering medication. Then we checked with Poison Control at the children's hospital in the city, and they confirmed our procedures. That's consistent with how we work, because we know the protocols for common things like that.

We have no lab to check blood levels of iron or Tylenol, so we had to transfer the baby on a medi-vac flight to the city. A nurse has to accompany the patients, and if we want a break, we try to get on that plane. The next day I had to go to another reservation in the satellite district, and wouldn't have been back in time, so another nurse went.

The blood values were not toxic and the baby returned the next morning by plane. We usually get reports on our medi-vacced patients, especially the trauma ones, and that adds to our knowledge base.

There are a fair number of married couples in the north. My wife and I are both nurses. The working setup is different because we know we can trust our backup person, and we know each other's strengths and weaknesses. It's a comfort knowing we'll never be stranded while on call.

If I've had a bad day with a lot of croupy kids or complaining mothers, I can express my feelings to my wife and get understanding feedback.

In the winter, depending on the ice, we snowmobile across the bay. Hockey is big and so is skating. Some isolated reservations are getting grants and building enclosed arenas, which provide a whole new vehicle to enjoy winter.

The men play hockey and the women play broomball. One place converted their arena into a roller skating rink. The available activities are gradually increasing. We enjoy dinners, bike riding, fishing, and boating. We socialize with the RCMP, many of whom are also married couples.

MAKE MY STAY
- R - R - R -

"When I was working as a public health nurse for the Saskatchewan government," reports Kelly, "I was asked to replace a nurse in one of the remote nursing stations."

I accepted, hoping for some excitement. The other nurse, in her eagerness to begin her Christmas holidays, gave me the scantiest of reports. She made home visits, she said, especially if there was a sick baby, but most patients came in to the station. And she was off.

The nursing station was on one corner of a large quadrangle, and the school was kitty-corner. On my first day there I was surprised to see fifteen smiling kids knocking at my door.

"Hi, how are you?" I said.

They stood there expectantly.

"What do I do with them?" I whispered to the housekeeper. "Obviously they're waiting for something."

"They're here for their vitamins." She showed me where they were stored and I handed them out.

Half an hour later more kids arrived, and again I dispensed vitamins. The housekeeper looked perplexed, but said nothing.

The next day, the same thing. Two groups of kids at my door. The housekeeper laughed so hard she cried. "These are the same kids," she spluttered, "coming to see the new nurse."

On the third day, the housekeeper shooed the kids away after their first visit. For a couple of days, they got double the goodies, a good joke on the new nurse.

PROFESSIONAL ISOLATION
- ℞ - ℞ - ℞ -

"For me, working with the Inuit population remains fascinating after ten years," says nurse Rochelle.

The north attracts people who don't follow the crowd, who want different life experiences. Recently, I had the privilege of working with a sixty-two-year-old nurse, who for some thirty years trained African women to be midwives. She's a nun, a sister of the African order.

Health and disease issues are changing here as a result of a change in lifestyle. For instance, ten years ago there was no sugar or jam for my toast, and there was no diabetes, high blood pressure, or heart problems. Now the grocery store has everything available that I can have down south. Videos and TV keep everyone far more sedentary than before.

I'm the only nurse working with natives and I train them to be quasi-nurses, while I function as a quasi-doctor. Such solo nursing, as it's called, brings up the interesting issue of professional isolation. In certain situations it would be beneficial to talk to another professional.

In this society, a male will phone us regarding any serious problems. Some of the ladies don't have enough confidence in themselves to make the call. For example, on the weekend a man called regarding a little boy who had a nasty laceration on his knee from playing with a piece of wood. The father was away, so the mother got the male neighbour to phone me.

Culturally, I feel in-between, because I am so immersed in the Inuit's culture. It was curious when I first began to realize that my own culture was disappearing in part. I speak Inuktituk in working conversation, like "Hi, my name is Rochelle, what's your name? I'm a nurse. Do you have pain?" Ordinary things. I can't understand everything, but I can get the gist of a conversation.

Nurses are treated as important people by the Inuit. The order of priority is God, Chief, and Head Nurse. The recognition we have here as professionals is a big reason why nurses come back to the north.

For example, one Monday morning as a mark of special consideration, a float plane was chartered especially for me to fly to a more northern vicinity that had no nurse at all.

The Chief asked if I would replace two community health representatives who were to be off for the summer. This was a satellite community of another community, so it was the first time they had a nurse. I was on call for a whole month.

I saw many grateful patients with a variety of medical problems. This little community had a detox centre, but no running water, no washrooms, and only one phone. Yes, this was in the nineties.

A teenager I had seen the previous week came in with a lacerated hand. We chatted as I took care to remove all the sand particles that were ground into his cut. Being a male teenager, he fainted. And this was the son of the Chief. I felt so bad and afraid, but I had no other professional to talk to. Solo nursing.

The surroundings are not always positive in the north because of the social problems and the physical environment. But it is important for any human being to be recognized for what they are doing. Down south, we're told only when we do something wrong, and if we do our work well, nobody notices.

Another time I flew to Baffin Island to pick up a newborn baby with pneumonia. They had chartered a 748, which is bigger than a twin-engine Otter, because of the long distance and the constant threat of weather on Baffin Island.

Many of the seats had been removed for cargo-carrying purposes. I was in this huge airplane with two pilots in the front, and an overall-garbed flight attendant who was prepared to serve Pepsi and peanuts. En route, the co-pilot invited me to sit up front with the pilot, while he chatted with the flight attendant.

I've been to Alaska and to the Yukon to see the icebergs, but the ones I saw on the way to Baffin Island were absolutely the most spectacular ones I ever saw in my life. And the pilot pointed out the mountains where a James Bond film was made. What an incredible flight.

Oftentimes in the north nurses don't want to go on these flights — they're sick or they don't want to risk crashing. Because I always loved going, I was called "the medi-vac woman." Whenever there was a flight, I was ready to go.

Another time a doctor came with me to insert a chest drain into a man who had shot himself. We picked him up in northern Quebec and flew to the nearest hospital, which was on Baffin Island.

The doctor knew about a beautiful crater in Quebec where a meteorite had landed years ago and made a perfectly round circle. On the way back he asked the pilot to show it to us. It was tremendously exciting. This African nurse was telling me she wants to see this very crater before she dies.

Everybody is affected by their environment, and the same is true up north. When a storm lasts for three days, we can't see the next house, and we've run out of milk, we have to be ingenious — and we need our neighbours.

On the weekend I was speaking with some teachers, and sometimes wish I had their lifestyle. At five o'clock their life is their own. They're never on call. When I was doing solo nursing, I was always on call. Now there's another nurse, so we're on call only one day out of two.

Often I just have time enough to recuperate. It's too demanding and I don't want to work full-time anymore. I have an apartment in the south of Quebec and that suits me just fine.

THE GOAT RAFFLE
- R - R - R -

Patsy loves nursing in northern British Columbia where she grew up. "We have beautiful summers here," she says. "We're in a valley so it's quite warm.

"There are about a thousand of us, counting the farming area. The people out here are tough."

We get everything from seizures to vehicle accidents in the clinic. The doctor sees up to twenty-five patients a day plus emergencies. There's no one here on nights or on the weekends. If someone is injured or if there's an accident, the RCMP call me or someone will come and pick me up.

Our clinic is too small. When we get an arrest or a major injury, it's terrible. I've had to climb over bodies to get to the other side of the bed for a certain piece of equipment. It gets pretty wild. We could use ropes from the ceiling to swing on.

We've had some sad summers, like the one where three of our teenagers were killed in separate accidents. Not one was drinking and driving, which was unusual. One was going to school on his motorcycle and got hit by a flatbed truck. He died of massive head injuries. Another was chopping trees with his friends, and a tree landed on him. The third was in a car that rolled and he flew out of the back seat, through the windshield.

People here look at health care differently. They swear by yucca tea for their arthritis and most of them refuse aspirin. If their blood pressure is high they eat celery. They will only take medication if the celery doesn't work.

The older people are tough and this rubs off on the youngsters. A teenager came in on a Monday morning with two partially collapsed lungs. She didn't call on the weekend because she didn't want to bother anyone. People are like that up here.

The nearest hospital is forty-five miles away, but it has no surgical facilities. The roads aren't that great to get there either. The road keeps sliding, and it may be closed for days at a time.

When I transferred a stroke patient recently, the ambulance driver was brand new and a wild driver. I hit the ceiling, flew over top of my patient and hit the wall, breaking the plexi-glass on the cupboard. But she keeps us all going at the clinic because she's so funny. Once she was in such a hurry she panicked and left without the other ambulance attendants. We saw them flagging her down on the road. She's starting to calm down a bit now.

We get the air ambulance for the critically ill, but it takes so long to get up here. For instance, a man was visiting friends in thirty-five degree below weather. On the way home, his vehicle broke down and he tried to walk back, but didn't make it.

The next morning some friends found his dog in an alleyway. The dog led them to him, but he was unconscious and hypothermic by this time. It took three and a half hours for the paramedics from southern BC to come in the air ambulance to pick him up.

Most of our murders stem from drinking parties. There's a fair amount of drinking in the north. The calls we get at night are always dreadful, and then we have to get up for the clinic in the morning. It's tiring because there are so many accidents.

One day a week we set aside certain hours for house calls, but we may see our palliative care people several times a week. In a little two-room cabin, with no power or phone, an older man with cancer lived.

"Watch out for the bears. There was one at the window this morning," he yelled out to me. I parked my vehicle by the doorstep, lined up my door with his, and ran in. But he was never afraid.

The elderly generally refuse to go into nursing homes because they've lived here all their lives. Some of their homes are filthy and I feel like having a shower afterward. One lady whose husband passed away refused to go to a nursing home, even though her memory was poor. When I went to see her the front door was frozen shut. I had to use the tire iron to beat the door in, and chip the ice away to shut it. She hadn't been able to go outside for days.

We do bereavement calls. The people appreciate our visits, but tend to overfeed us. Many are good friends. It's a different environment here.

Our elderly people really are exceptionally active. I see one eighty-year-old man down in the ditch with his horses, riding with his granddaughters or chopping wood. He only comes to the clinic if he's been trampled by his bull. He makes me feel like one of these city sludge people.

The community is quite healthy and enjoys the lifestyle program. They get into walking programs because they get T-shirts and trips and points, and various other incentives.

We have one grocery store, a garage, and a gas station in town. In the middle is a huge up-to-date fitness centre. That's kind of odd, considering we don't even have a ladies' clothing store. Interesting community that way.

We look after animals as well as people. I love animals and right now I'm training my husky-wolf dog team to pull a sleigh. I took an animal sciences course because we get a lot of veterinarian calls. Technically, we can't do them, but the nearest vet is forty-five miles away and sometimes asks us to help. I sewed a newborn pig's ear on when the momma pig accidentally ripped it off with her foot. I took the costs for the suture and local anesthetic out of our coffee fund, because we don't charge for this kind of work.

Another time I started an IV on a cat. When the doctor and I got out to the farm, she was as cold as stone, seizuring, and had aspirated. She was pregnant and we decided she must be calcium deficient. We gave her some Ventolin, calcium, and an antibiotic, and she picked right up. I brought her home with me that night to keep an eye on her and to keep her warm. By morning she had fully recovered.

Every year we have a Goat Raffle in town. You buy tickets for somebody you hate, and if they win, they get the goat. The tickets sell really well and are available at the clinic. This is where Coconut, one of my three goats, came from. The man who won her was going to shoot her, so I brought her home. Coconut, Jenny, and Daisy mow our three-acre lawn in no time. It used to take eighteen hours by hand.

In the summer there are so many moose and elk we have to drive slowly. Almost everyone in town has hit a deer. One day I counted four hundred deer on the way in to town. Or we come across herds of cows on the road.

I hit a horse on the way to work one day, and did ten thousand dollars worth of damage to my truck. I wasn't injured too badly, but the horse died. I should open up a road kill restaurant.

LIFE WITH DIGNITY
– ꝶ – ꝶ – ꝶ –

"The first medical evacuation I did in the Northwest Territories," says nurse Florence, *"greatly affected my feeling*

of what was happening with the Inuit in the north, and what they had to contend with."

I was called to bring out an older Inuit man who lived up on Victoria Island in the Arctic. The Roman Catholic priest, who was the lay dispenser there, phoned out. He thought the old fellow had had a heart attack. I had to go and bring him back to our hospital for treatment.

I flew up in the back of a Hercules that happened to be going up with a load of fuel. The pilot, co-pilot, and I left early on a winter's evening. There were no seats. The entire plane was loaded with drums of gasoline and I had to sit on the floor in the back, where it was freezing cold. After the three hour flight, the plan was to unload the gasoline and load up again with empty drums.

We were met there by the R.C. priest who led me to the igloo. We crawled in through the entrance and there, in the corner, was a man laying on caribou furs. His daughter sat beside him. It was as warm as toast with a seal oil lamp burning. I felt the sense of a complete family unit and that they were happy with the way things were.

The priest came in and we began the interviewing. It took half an hour of questioning back and forth. In English, I told the priest what I wanted to know, and the priest interpreted it in Inuktuk to the girl. She then spoke in Inuktuk to her father. I asked the priest why he didn't speak directly to the father. He told me the father had told him earlier that he was too ill and preferred to leave it up to his daughter.

The man's pulse was slow, his blood pressure was high, and he was breathing shallowly. He had no clamminess or fever. He didn't say much. The priest thought it was a heart attack, but I had no way of determining what was wrong with him and I had no medications. There was little I could do except bring him out.

By this time the pilots had finished unloading their fuel and were ready to leave. One of them came up to the entrance of the igloo to see if we were ready. They wanted to figure out where they were going to put the stretcher that I had brought with me on the plane.

But the old man did not want to come. A lot of the Inuit had been sent out with tuberculosis in the 1950s and never returned, and this is what happened to his wife. They didn't know what had happened to her, or whether she was still alive or not. There had been no communication and there seemed to be no way for them to get information. "If I'm going to die," he said, "I want to die in my own home."

It was so emotional. He started crying and the daughter was crying, and before we finished, I was crying too. It was then that I learned the real reason for our four-way conversation. The old man was so adamant about not coming out that he refused to speak to the priest when he discovered his intention of sending him out. Consequently the priest had to speak through the daughter.

Something came over me at that point and I said, "That's fine. He doesn't have to come out. We won't take him."

The priest was upset, but I said, "If this man wants to stay here, I can't in all consciousness take him out."

I told the priest what I thought the daughter should do to keep her father comfortable. Unless he changed his mind, he could stay in his own home.

I nearly froze to death on the way home. The empty gas drums were thumping around on the floor, and I sat on my sleeping bag, shivering, thinking I had failed my first medi-vac.

We got home at four in the morning. I was almost afraid to go to work a few hours later and admit I hadn't brought my patient out. The nurse-in-charge wanted to know all the details and was empathetic. We discussed it at some length and she agreed I had done the right thing.

The doctor said, "That's fine. If he wouldn't come, he wouldn't come," but he was business-like about it and showed no real understanding. There were no repercussions.

It's one of the things that over the years has stuck in my mind. I had a different attitude from that time on, and when we went out to do our clinics and worked with the Dene Indians in their villages, I felt humble about going into their homes. I hoped we could help them without changing their culture, their feelings

about health, or the way they looked after their own
people.

NOT ME
- ₱ - ₱ - ₱ -

*In Manitoba, Liz, like any good nurse, knows that
what patients say can be far removed from what the real
problem is.*

We see a lot of solvent abuse up here. A mother
of six came in complaining of pain in her lower back and
abdomen after falling down a flight of stairs. She said
she had been drinking hair spray for two weeks.

After a cursory examination I suspected she was
pregnant and in labour.

"Is it possible that you're pregnant?" I asked.

"Not me," she said. "Definitely not."

"Let's just check you out and be certain."

Sure enough, she was in labour, about three to
four centimetres dilated. I moved her into the obstetrics
room across the hall for observation, while she kept
insisting she wasn't pregnant. She hurt herself when she
fell, why couldn't I understand that.

Although she remained relatively comfortable, I
decided to examine her once more. The other nurse in
the room wasn't gloved yet.

I looked and oh goodness, there was something
coming out — the baby was crowning. The next minute

the membrane went pphhhhhttttt! up my arm and all over me from my neck down. We had long green isolation gowns on, but it was still kind of gross.

I held the baby's head as it came out and checked for the cord, while the other nurse suctioned the baby. The mother gave a loud "Nnnggggppp," wiggled a bit, and the baby popped out.

The baby took three minutes to breathe properly because the mother had abused solvents and alcohol throughout the pregnancy — the sniff and drinking again. I was so scared about this tiny girl because her apgar rating was low, and it didn't look too good there for a while.

I saw a pool of blood and thought I better get the placenta delivered. I pulled on the cord with slight traction and it came out intact.

Within a short time the baby improved and turned out to be just fine. I wanted the mother to name her baby after me, because I had been so worried about her, but she wouldn't and I was upset.

THE LAST PATROL
- R - R - R -

Lee, a nurse in the Northwest Territories, concludes that today's current business concepts concern self-managing work teams.

This is familiar to Lee, who was nurse-in-charge on the last medical patrol of the C.D. Howe, an ice-breaker in the high Arctic. "We were thrown together from June until

October," she says, *"and we became a team in short order for the sake of our patients."*

The *C.D. Howe* operated like a hospital for National Health and Welfare, and visited the out-settlements in the high Arctic. One terrible experience sticks out in my mind, but it's balanced by other positive ones.

Twenty people were on board, the crew plus the medical team, which was selected from all over Canada — physicians, dentists, a dental assistant, an epidemiologist, an x-ray technician, a researcher, RNs, and an RNA.

When we left I was a regional nursing officer in the Yukon. To my horror, I learned that a physician who was impossible to work with was also going. Gritting my teeth, I felt that one of us would not return.

We provisioned in Montreal and Quebec City, and embarked from the shores of northern Quebec. First we voyaged to Hudson's Bay, then north to Baffin Island. From there, we navigated through to our most northerly destination, Grise Fiord on Ellesmere Island.

The settlements knew exactly when the ice-breaker was coming, because the helicopter on board flew ahead and gave them twenty-four hour advance notice, and apprised them of any delays when we got stuck in the ice.

Because the Inuit were scattered all over in summer camps, we functioned like a community health van. The barge cruised to the mainland, filled up with prospective patients, and returned to the ship.

We zeroed in on preventative medicine and immunizations, checking the nomadic peoples. Two Inuit interpreters on board fought the language barrier for us.

We worked until we were finished, and that often meant going from four in the morning until sometime the next day. After the people were returned on the barge we packed up and left.

Although I was familiar with the aboriginal culture in the Yukon, I didn't have a good working knowledge of the Inuit culture. I had no idea of their customs, but as my understanding of them gradually grew I found them to be fascinating.

They brought a dead infant to the ship. According to their culture, it was permissible to throw a female into the sea, if a male was desired. Because this practice was becoming less acceptable, we were asked to determine whether this baby was stillborn or alive when thrown into the sea.

The sea provided the method of disposal. Normally, because of frigid temperatures, they would have to wait until the land thawed enough to bury their dead.

I gritted my teeth while we did the autopsy on the tiny sea-washed infant. I was appalled at such a procedure being performed on one so small, and the terrible memory remains. We determined that the baby probably was stillborn.

Afterward, the doctor gave non-smoking me one of his hateful cigars. I had about five puffs on this smelly thing as a method of coping with what I had just seen.

We had to perform an emergency appendectomy on a little boy with a ruptured appendix. There was no surgeon on board and I had always hated the operating room. Nonetheless, one of the physicians and I set up an OR.

It looked like something from a Ding Bat calender and was located at the rear of the ship, under the helicopter deck. Every time the helicopter took off or landed, all the instruments and tables in the OR vibrated. Between us, we successfully removed the boy's appendix and drained his abdomen.

We nursed him on board ship until he was healthy enough to be flown back to his village. In all, we had to perform surgery three times, so our surgical skills increased dramatically.

We were totally dependent on one another, and initially there was friction. The physician I disliked told me he too thought only one of us would return. However, with the intensity of team development, we became good friends.

As the daylight hours decreased, our affection for the ship increased. We loved to see the lights of the ship riding at anchor as we returned from the villages on the darkened barge. The aroma of delicious meals wafted over the waves in salutation. We became part of the ship, and the ship was our home in every sense.

We de-provisioned in Frobisher Bay, and once emptied, made our way back down the coast of Labrador. In Quebec, we disembarked and made our separate ways back home, richer by far for the unique experience.

TEN

CHALK IT UP TO EXPERIENCE
- ℞ - ℞ - ℞ -

To a great experience one thing is essential,
an experiencing nature.
Walter Bagehot, 1826-1877

Canadian nurses undergo a great variety of encounters in their professional adventures. Nestled amongst them are the familiar options of "damned if you do and damned if you don't," as well as the placement of the proverbial foot in the mouth from time to time.

One shocking way in which society is changing is reflected in the increasing awareness of violence. For those in the nursing profession, this may mean attending to clashes between patients or dealing with violence aimed directly at the nurse.

A bit of humour, a bit of tragedy, a bit of irony. What is there to say? All shifts eventually come to an end.

Chalk it up to experience.

Lillian R. Tymchuk, RN

LOVE THY NEIGHBOUR
- ℞ - ℞ - ℞ -

"If ever there was a major pain in the butt," says Lucy from her spinal cord floor, "it was Smittie, a quadriplegic and ostensibly the worst patient I ever had." Lucy is one of 100,937 nurses in Ontario.

On evenings, we heard a huge commotion down the hall, and we knew it was coming from Smittie's room.

Smittie raised a lot of hell for an eighteen-year-old, threatening his buds unless they brought forbidden drugs and alcohol in for him, yelling and screaming at staff if his needs and wants weren't immediately attended to, blaming other patients for taking up the nurses' time, complaining about the meals, physio, his wheelchair, his showers, his bowel routine, his clothes, the TV programs, the weather, the movies, and his catheterization times, to name a few. Smittie was paralyzed from the neck down. He ignored all positive intervention attempts.

Now it sounded like he was in trouble. Should we walk quickly or should we walk slowly? Do we want to help this patient or do we want to ignore him?

We walked down the hall — at a medium pace — to his room and peeked in. Hal, a young paraplegic in his wheelchair, was doing his utmost to strangle Smittie, who by this time was half in bed and half out.

Such a confrontation wasn't totally unexpected, because Smittie mercilessly taunted Hal, trying to ignite his short fuse. Smittie was goading him on to strangle him, to kill him.

"You haven't got the balls to kill me, you creep. You're nothing but a wussie."

I have to admit the thought briefly crossed my mind that the floor would be so peaceful without Smittie. Do we pull Hal away or do we let him do it? Which professional nursing theory would best suit this situation?

Hal clutched Smittie by the throat with his left hand and his right one gripped the black rubber tire of his locked wheelchair. He squeezed both hands so tightly his knuckles whitened and perspiration dripped from his forehead. Smittie's useless arms dangled lifelessly at his side, but his eyes widened in a beet-red face. We separated them with great difficulty because of the enormous strength in Hal's arms — he lifted weights and worked with horses before his accident.

I realized if he had chosen to kill Smittie he could have done so. But he didn't want to, and the only way to save face was for him to allow us to separate them. He wanted to be able to tell Smittie, "I would've killed you if they didn't pull me off."

Smittie called me everything under the sun, so I decided to file charges against him. I called the hospital administrator and the nurse on call, to inform them. I could see no valid reason to put up with this garbage.

The administrator had not been aware what we, as nurses, were putting up with. He came in and read Smittie the riot act. He told him this behaviour was to STOP NOW or he would find himself living on the street; he'd be thrown out. That was the last problem we had ever with Smittie.

BIG BLUNDER
- R - R - R -

Pediatric nurse Charlotte explains her mistake in Manitoba thus: "It was my fourth night. This proves I wasn't completely awake."

There were so many young girls admitted with anorexia and bulimia they were spread throughout the entire hospital. That's how we ended up with Annie on our peds floor.

It was 8:00 P.M., the beginning of a twelve-hour night shift. I wasn't feeling so hot. I was dog tired and not clicking in to things. Annie was sitting on the bed watching TV when we made rounds.

"Do you need anything?" I asked her.

"No."

"Do you want a VCR to watch movies?"

"No, I'm watching TV tonight."

"What are you watching?"

"Roseanne."

"She looks great, doesn't she. She's lost so much weight."

I was halfway down the hall before I realized what I said. Nurse, you made a faux pas.

THE CAN
– ₨ – ₨ – ₨ –

"When I first came to the Northwest Territories," says nurse Sherry, *"our health unit did all the evacuations out of the high Arctic and the whole western Arctic, a tremendously large area.*

"There were thirty Armed Forces families with all their kids and dogs living in the hotel for two months before the housing was ready for us."

In the nursing station there weren't any phones. I was informed via ham radio concerning a flight to the high Arctic to evacuate a patient.

Where I was going there was no nursing station. Five adults and three children peopled a little northern community. It took two days of travelling in a canoe for two men to reach the closest settlement with a ham radio. It was from there that we received the message.

I had never flown in a small plane before and didn't realize there was no bathroom on board. I drank cup after cup of steaming hot coffee to calm my jittery nerves. The pilot and I flew over a beautiful but barren land. From the air everything looked the same — there were no villages or landmarks of any kind for hundreds of miles.

We approached an area where people were living in the middle of nowhere. We landed on floats, a strange sensation for the uninitiated, and almost got blown away by a wild, angry wind. In the vastness of the landscape there was not one tree.

My first priority was to see the patient, but after all that coffee, I was in such agony to get to a bathroom I couldn't focus on anything else. The people there didn't speak English and I wondered what to do. The best I could come up with was to indicate drinking from a cup and then squatting. They took me to a little shed with a pail.

I was ready to see my patient now. A young man, barely out of his teens, was curled up on a bed, moaning. His knees were drawn up and perspiration poured from his flushed face.

I gave him Demerol and started an IV. We flew him to the city where he had surgery for a perforated appendix. This handsome young man was stoic throughout his rough ordeal, and so appreciative of his care. I felt in my heart that the courage shown by the Inuit could overcome the demands of an awe-inspiring but cruel land.

PERPLEXED PILOT
- R - R - R -

"My patient was hauling logs when he fractured his pelvis in a dog team accident," says Quebec nurse Lucille. "How could I tell him we were lost?"

Our small Quebec hospital was on the Gulf of St. Lawrence and I was transferring a patient with the Grenfell mission to northern Newfoundland. It was a short trip, less than an hour, so I didn't take much equipment with me.

The pilot was a nice chap. He spoke English to me and French to his base via radio. My patient was relatively comfortable during the flight, and as we neared our destination flying over the straits, the pilot said, "We'll land on the airstrip."

"Not here we won't," I said. "This isn't the right place." I had flown on a similar transfer once before and what I saw was not familiar.

"Where are we?" the pilot asked. Talk about inspiring confidence.

"Where are we?" he repeated.

"I have no idea."

"I'm out of fuel. I'll have to come down on the sea ice."

"Get down then," I said.

We circled around until we found a harbour. The landing was rough because the sea ice was so bumpy, being near the end of winter. My patient was in the back on a back board, rattling around with his poor fractured pelvis.

All the local people ran out when we landed, chattering away. It's not every day a plane arrives on the sea with a pilot and a nurse.

"Do you know what they're saying?" the bewildered pilot asked.

I wasn't used to the Newfoundland accent either. So there was the pilot with his French accent, and me with my Scottish one.

"First of all," I said, "tell us where we are."

They told us. "Is there a nursing station or any medical facility close by?" I asked hopefully.

"Sure, nurse, there's a nursing station thirty miles down the road."

"Do you have an ambulance or any kind of vehicle?"

"There's the school bus."

"What's the road like?"

"It's pretty rough, nurse."

"Well, forget it," I said, "I can't have my patient clattering around on a rough road."

One of the older couples kindly said, "You can come to our house. We'll look after you until you can get away."

It was getting too dark to fly anyway, and before I could say "Winkie," these wonderful people were helping us.

They had to remove the front door of the house to get my patient in on his back board. The lady made us feel most welcome and made an appetizing supper.

I didn't have pain killers with me because I had given my patient something for pain just before we left, and didn't anticipate needing any more before we landed. I phoned the nursing station, and unbelievably a doctor was there.

"I'll come up and bring some medication for you," he said amiably enough after I explained my predicament. He drove the thirty miles in an antiquated vehicle, delivered the analgesics, and left.

I was really annoyed with the pilot because he shouldn't have lost his way in the first place. When I called the hospital and told them where we were, they couldn't believe it.

I advised the pilot to get some sleep. "I'll get you up in the morning to check the weather," I said.

The weather was always going in and out up there — it was terrible. True to my word I woke him up in the early dawn.

"But nurse," he whined, "it's still dark. We can't even see the weather."

"I don't care. You get on the radio and you find out."

Reluctantly, he called the hospital and a supervisor said, "Just wait now till I look out the window." A moment later she said, "It's too dark to see anything."

The pilot said, "I know it's dark, but just give me any old weather forecast to get this nurse off my back."

He relayed the message that a storm was coming our way.

"I don't care. We're going in the air now," I told him.

At six in the morning, it was only starting to get light, but I felt my poor patient had gone through enough already. From nowhere men appeared to help us, and I gathered my things together. Some kind soul there gave us enough AV gas for the flight. Carrying my patient to the plane was a struggle, but we couldn't put him on a snowmobile. These wonderful people helped us load him into the plane, and we prepared to take off.

The anxious pilot turned around to face me. "I've got no light on my control panel," he said apprehensively.

By this time I was fit to be tied. "Do you have a flashlight?" I snarled. "Give it to me. I'll shine the flashlight, and you check the controls. We're leaving now!"

"Okay nurse."

As it turned out, we were only off course by ten minutes the night before, but it was over the mountains, and I don't know if he had enough fuel anyway.

Thankfully there was little turbulence to mar our flight. As we flew over the harbour, we could see the Simon Fraser ice-breakers had been up the night before, and chewed up all the harbour ice.

"This is terrific," I said. "Where do we land now?"

Our plane could land on either wheels or skis. The pilot found one square inch of ice and landed on the skis.

"You'd better be quick," he warned, "because I think the weather's coming down."

A waiting ambulance drove us to the nearby hospital, where I quickly settled my tired patient. I couldn't have been gone more than fifteen or twenty minutes.

Whenever a plane came over the Straits of Belle Isle, they usually loaded it up with doctors and nurses and whoever else for the return flight. When I got back there were all these doctors from the Grenfell Mission lined up to go back. We boarded and took off.

After a few brief moments in the air I felt the plane turning around.

"Are you lost again?" I demanded.

"The weather's come down," the pilot said. "I can't see over the straits."

We returned to Newfoundland and it was five days before I could get back home to Quebec.

CERTIFIABLE
- R - R - R -

"The Public Health Department referred Claudia to Mental Health, and asked us to do an assessment on her," explains nurse Sarah in Prince Edward Island.

Claudia was a senior citizen with diabetes, about twice the size of her husband. They lived in a senior citizens' complex out in the country.

The public health nurses were concerned. When they made their regular visits they felt she was often paranoid, that some things she said weren't true. At other times she presented as being perfectly lucid. But there were persistent stories about her beating up on her husband.

I was assigned to do the assessment and made a home visit. After I explained why I had come she seemed delighted to see me. She was pleasant, alert, oriented, and denied any problems in terms of her relationship with her husband. The husband also denied any problems.

Before my second visit, Claudia called to make sure I was coming. Things were progressing smoothly. On my third visit I went into the living room as usual.

"Oh, you're the nurse," Claudia said. "I never liked any of you. You've been trying to steal my husband for the last ten years."

She picked up a big brass lamp with a beige shade and hurled it with all her might. She missed her moving target.

Because no doctor had seen her we couldn't certify her. It took a week and a half to get her admitted. Her frightened husband wouldn't call us. We found out later she locked him out at night, and he slept in a little laundry room without a door. Claudia also accused the lady next door of sleeping with her husband and other delusional things.

Twice I arranged for her to go into the emergency department. I told the doctors she would present as fairly lucid initially. "If you want to find the psychosis," I advised, "you have to keep her for at least an hour."

Both times the doctor on call saw her, checked her diabetes, said there was nothing wrong and sent her home. When Claudia started beating her husband up again, the neighbours called the Mounties and she was certified and admitted to the psychiatric floor.

CORNED BEEF AND CABBAGE
- ℞ - ℞ - ℞ -

Nurse Helen says, "We look after the frail, elderly adults who are admitted to the infirmary in New Brunswick. They are combatting the aging process, medical illness, and a superimposed psychiatric problem."

As in any psychiatric facility we have a certain number of male staff members, but contrary to what the general public may think, we do not have big burly men to do our bidding, so we, as women, won't have to do anything physically taxing.

One day I proceeded to pivot Maxwell, one of my patients, out of his bed and into a special geri-chair. I'm five foot one and he's at least six foot four, so I'm already at a disadvantage. He has femurs that are longer than my entire body, and he probably weighs a couple of hundred pounds, even in his debilitated arthritic state.

I counted "One-Two-Three" to get him into a standing position, and out of the corner of my eye I could see Nathan, one of our other gentlemen — a feeble, declining man suffering from a manic-depressive disorder which did not abate in his declining years. He raised his dinner tray with both hands and swung it around to one side.

"Whatever you do, Nathan," I pleaded, "whatever you do, don't throw the tray. I beg you, DON'T THROW THE TRAY."

He looked at me and set the tray back on his bedside table. In a heartbeat, he picked up his dinner plate full of corned beef and cabbage, took aim, and pitched it straight at me and Maxwell.

Now that corned beef and cabbage, as is wont to do with Murphy's Law, landed right under Maxwell's arthritic feet. He starting to slip and slide in the cabbage.

"Timber," I called out. "TIMBER."

How I managed to get Maxwell into the geri-chair, albeit a little lop-sided, I'll never know. But at least he wasn't on the floor and he didn't fall on top of me.

I straightened him up and cleaned the cabbage up with a bath towel. Nathan was humming.

"You had to do it, Nathan, didn't you? You had to do it."

"Nothing to do with me, hum-hum."

He shook his strawberry Pro-drink milkshake so violently it exploded in his face.

"Bien agiter," he said, throwing the carton at me.

FIRST COURSE — MURDER
- R - R - R -

Nurse Cathy had to change restaurants as a result of one shift in her Saskatchewan emergency department.

Two ambulance attendants brought a beautiful young woman in, unconscious. They said the husband said he found her lying in bed when he got home from work and called for help.

She died within minutes. It was considered to have been a suicide. An overdose. A heartbroken husband arrived shortly after with two bewildered little kids in tow. He was a well-known businessman, a chef in his own popular restaurant. All the nurses knew him well.

Right out of the blue I got a subpoena. The police had charged him with murder. I had to testify as an emergency nurse about the condition of his wife when she was brought in, knowing that he was sitting there. Talk about an uncomfortable situation.

He got off, but eighty percent of everyone who had anything to do with the case, felt he was responsible for her death. I wasn't taking any chances — I changed restaurants.

I see him around all the time, and that doesn't help. We see these people at their absolute worst, and then we run into them in the grocery store or in the shopping mall.

They remember us as the nurse and our face is going to be sticking right in their brain. For the one nurse they see, there are hundreds of patients we see. Sometimes it's hard to put a face and a story together. I don't want to say the wrong thing like, "How is your brother?" and find out he was the one brought in DOA.

Another big concern is confidentiality. I live in a small town and people phone me and say, "Milly went to the hospital today. What's wrong with her?"

I constantly have to say, "I'm sorry, if you want to find out about Milly, you have to phone her husband. It's not up to me to say."

When I see them downtown, they give me that "you bitch" look. It goes with the territory.

WARM AND DEAD
- R - R - R -

"In the Yukon, you have to be warm and dead before you're pronounced dead." This ironic statement comes from nurse Terry.

In the north, people die from hypothermia, so if somebody is found dead in the snow we have to warm them up before the doctor can officially pronounce them dead. The warming up process may take up to five hours, especially if someone comes in stiff as a board.

One Sunday night I was supervising as well as working in emergency. We got a call about a man caught in an avalanche that occurred quite a distance away. From the time we dispatched a helicopter manned by two doctors, and they picked him up, he had been frozen for approximately four and a half hours.

On the return flight one of the doctors called in from the helicopter saying they were about to land in the parking lot. This area was not designed for helicopter landings, and there was the obvious danger of cars during evening visiting hours.

I phoned our ambulance drivers who have their own area right beside the parking lot. "The helicopter is landing on the parking lot right now. Get all the vehicles out and make sure no visitors come anywhere near."

"You got it."

Emergency was already wild because we had four teenagers who had been covered by mounds of snow from another avalanche. We've been getting more avalanches lately because people are going out to the Pass on skidoos, and snowboarding and telemarking in dangerous areas, and they don't always know how to read the snow.

Minutes later I received yet another phone call from the ambulance dispatcher. An airplane with twenty-five people on board had radioed in, saying they didn't know if the landing wheels had come out or not, so a belly landing was a very real possibility. Anticipating a crash, the ambulance personnel had to tear off for the airport.

I looked out the emergency window and my heart raced a hundred miles a minute. The helicopter was hovering overhead, while a mini-van pulled in under it. How disaster was averted, I'll never know.

My guardian angel must have been working overtime that evening, because at the airport, the landing wheels and the plane came down safely at the last second. Emergency was already far too busy to handle another twenty-five victims from a plane crash.

Then, in rushed the doctors with the hypothermic man from the avalanche. No heart rate, but they had been doing continuous CPR for hours.

We rushed him downstairs to physio to warm him up in the large hubbard tank. Believe me, he was stiff as a board. We couldn't even get an IV into him until we warmed him up a bit. ICU was full, so we couldn't put him there, and emerg was full. I was running all over trying to get more staff to help. I had to call in three other nurses plus a doctor.

It was a horrendous night for everybody involved. It took three rotating ambulance people to perform constant CPR. We had our crash cart available, and we were prepared to dry him immediately if there was any change.

Once we got him to a certain temperature we took him out of the hubbard tank and put him on the cardiac monitor. Often these patients go into ventricular fibrillation as they warm up, and we had to be ready with staff and equipment.

Four hours after he arrived we got the biggest shock of all — we started getting a rhythm on the cardiac monitor. Everybody stopped. What do we do if we bring him back to life?

We had worked on him for hours, but when we got this heart beat, we wondered what we had done. We just wanted to get him to the point where we could pronounce him dead.

In the end, the heart beat was just a fluke. He had been dead from the get go. That was our shift from Hell.

IF I CLOSE MY EYES
- ℞ - ℞ - ℞ -

Sandy, a nurse from Ontario, works in Saudi Arabia. "Life here is totally different from home," she says, "but the work is the same except we work a forty-four hour week."

The hospital and our living quarters are part of a military base compound. We have to show our ID pass every time we leave the area and there is a midnight curfew.

The cafeteria is segregated — the men eat downstairs and we women eat upstairs in a separate room, although we all work together on the nursing floors. When we go out to eat, there are separate sections of the restaurant reserved for women and married couples.

I've met several nurses with whom I socialize, if you can call it that. There isn't much to do unless you're sports-minded, which I'm not. Some of the nurses who have been here for a long time manage to keep busy socially. The American and French compounds often have parties and invite nurses for the weekend.

There's a recreation centre on my compound with a swimming pool, and a video room which plays videos most of the day. I don't have a radio or TV, and rarely read any newspapers, so I feel isolated.

Because of a rigid adherence to Islam, the sexes are strictly segregated in public and women are not allowed to drive. We have to follow Moslem rules and regulations, which means we cannot talk to men on the street or in the shops. We have to wear a long black cloak called an *abaya* over our clothes, like the Moslem women do.

Right now we're being harassed in the downtown shops to wear a scarf and cover over our heads. So far all the Westerners and foreign women are refusing, but this might change as the religious leaders, or *mutawa*, march up and down the streets carrying a stick. When they see us they try to frighten or harass us into covering our heads. They have been known to occasionally strike a woman to get their point across. Wearing a covering will be unpleasant in the summertime, when it gets to be forty degrees C.

The next thing you know we'll have to wear a veil and cover our faces, but when that happens, I plan on leaving this country. There are many places here where that is already a rule.

It's going to be a funny Christmas as we are not officially allowed to celebrate at work, and of course the downtown shops will not be decorated for the holidays. My regular days off happen to fall over Christmas. I'll try to phone home, but I imagine the lines will be tied up.

I work on a chronic male floor with twenty-five patients. I was surprised to see such a large number of major car accidents here in Saudi Arabia. There are many permanently disabled young men on my floor.

Most of them require total care — that means feeding and changing diapers all shift long. There's a lot of heavy lifting and my back has been aching. I don't know if I'll last another six months or not.

On my days off I go with my friends to the downtown area and look around the shops and usually go to a restaurant for a meal. There are only two restaurants we go to, so the food is getting quite monotonous. I can hardly wait to get home for some good homemade food or go out for Chinese food. Even a Wendy's hamburger sounds good. My sister-in-law makes a terrific lasagna and if I close my eyes, I can taste it.

WORMS
– ℞ – ℞ – ℞ –

"The perils of eating improperly cooked fish should not be underestimated." That's the opinion of nurse Yolanda, who loves nursing in a clinic in Manitoba.

An anxious-looking man in the waiting room beckoned to me.

"I've got to see the doctor right away." A tone of urgency marked his voice.

"What seems to be the problem?"

"My asshole fell out. I have to speak to the doctor."

"Come with me." I took the man into an examining room.

"What can I do for you?" the doctor asked.

"My asshole fell out."

"Take a seat. I'll be right with you."

"I can't sit. My asshole fell out."

After a short break I re-entered the examining room. The doctor had ascertained that this man had been eating improperly cooked fish, according to the medical notes on the chart.

The man had two tapeworms hanging out of his bum. The gloved doctor was trying to roll them up on a Q-tip.

"Take a pair of gloves and start rolling," he suggested.

The doctor continued yanking and rolling the worms while I grabbed some gloves. He was getting quite a bit of them out, but the worms were segmented, and kept breaking and sliding back in.

He grabbed the man's butt cheeks and pulled them apart.

"GET 'EM, GET 'EM," he screamed, but I heard a "SSSssssssssst," and they slid right back in.

The doctor was devastated. The worms disappeared and he had wanted more to send to the lab. He was still holding the man's cheeks apart. "They're gone," he said sadly.

"No place like home," I muttered under my breath.

The doctor gave me a look. "You're sick," he said, and left the room.

I asked the man to wait for his medication, but he left. So there's a man walking around the north with two worms that he got from eating uncooked fish. He must have thought he was cured.

Lillian R. Tymchuk, RN

THERE'S A HELICOPTER ON MY DIAMOND
- ₿ - ₿ - ₿ -

As much as Bonnie loves sports, this athletic nurse loves nursing on her little island in BC even more — most times. "It's ironic the way some things work out," she says.

I hated to miss playing baseball with my friends this particular evening, but I had to work. This game was our equivalent to the World Series.

An hour into my shift I got a call from the American Coast Guard. They asked how big a helicopter our heli-pad was geared for.

They had a sick person on board ship that they were concerned about. People from all over the world are on these freighters and the concerns are generally for infections or contagious diseases. They wanted to fly this person in via helicopter, but our heli-pad was much too small.

When we determined just how large the American helicopter was, we promptly cancelled the ball game and cleared the diamond. The huge helicopter landed safely on the ball diamond.

After an admission of short duration, the patient steadily improved and was discharged. Luckily, the ball game was rescheduled for one of my days off.

GROSS ME OUT, MAN
- R - R - R -

"We don't have as many drug addicts as a large city hospital, but we see our share of them demanding narcotics," says Alberta nurse Candy. *"This is the grossest experience I've had as a nurse."*

One night there were three of us working and I was in charge. At 2:00 A.M. I heard some unfamiliar noises in the back.

Karen was a well-experienced nurse known for keeping her cool. She stormed up the hall exasperated.

"Candy," she said, "you won't believe what's going on out there."

An RCMP car was parked outside the entrance of the emergency department. Officers and ambulance attendants milled about. I could see the RCMP car bouncing up and down. All the windows were fogged in, and I could barely make out a young man in the back seat.

He was eighteen, a service station attendant. A transient who got a summer job. He was picked up in the back of the hotel running around naked, screaming and yelling and swearing, and doing all manner of rude things to his body.

The staff and residents in the hotel were hanging out of their windows and balconies watching this spectacle. The RCMP officer was a young woman and she managed to bring him in to us in the back of her car.

He was totally spaced out on acid. He took something like eleven hits of acid at once, he and a buddy. The buddy was so scared he took off into the forest behind the hotel.

This boy was totally gone. He stripped all his clothes off and was masturbating. He was voiding. He was defecating. He lost all control.

We couldn't remove him from of the car. He was like one of those super balls that keep bouncing forever.

He continued doing all these grotesque things and he was yelling and screaming and all of a sudden he would slap his face up against the window, and it was like he was a trapped animal, like he wasn't human.

He yelled out numbers, "One-two-three-four-five-six-seven-eight-nine-ten," really fast, and then he yelled out colours, "Blue-red-white-orange-yellow-purple." I think this is normal behaviour with acid.

He calmed down for a while and then he escalated again, yelling out numbers and colours. If he saw one of the RCMP officers go by, he'd holler out, "PIG-PIG-PIG-PIG-PIG," followed by a string of profanity. It was absolutely gross.

They wanted to take him out of the car and I said, "No way! You can't take him out of the car. He's not safe. Where are we going to put him? We can't put him in a room. We can't tie him down."

The car seemed to be the safest place for him because the roof and the seats were padded. The windows were a problem, but at least he was contained.

I called the doctor on call and she was furious. It was the last thing she wanted to deal with. She wasn't in the hospital and the doctors only want to come in for emergencies. We made her come in anyway.

In a way, it was an emergency, but what could we do? We didn't know what he had taken. They tracked his buddy down, but he didn't know what type of acid they had taken. He said they did drugs all the time. We couldn't begin to sort out the possible combinations of drugs he could have taken. We just had to let him come down.

We decided to give him some Ativan. If we could settle him down long enough to put it into his mouth, hopefully it would calm him down.

The only person who could get close to him was one of the EMTs, an emergency medical technician. He had an excellent manner and was able to get this kid to sit in the front seat and open the window a bit. His goal was to put his hand through the open window and deposit the medication into this kid's mouth.

During several attempts, the kid lost it and clawed at the window like a wild animal trying to escape. He was totally slimed with vomit, urine, and feces. The energy he was releasing was unimaginable. The only good thing was that the car was so fogged up because of body heat and body fluids that we couldn't see everything he was doing. It was like a steam bath in there.

Finally the EMT gave him the Ativan. He sat in the car for hours until he chilled out enough to be taken to the police rubber room.

Technically, he was fine the next day. He left the police station and that was the end of it. Heaven knows how many brain cells he had left. We had no follow-up because he left town, like most of our younger transients do.

I was grossed out for a long time, but I wish we had filmed it. This is what we need to show to school kids.

AYE OR NAY
- ₽ - ₽ - ₽ -

"At break-up and freeze-up in the Northwest Territories, we flew in by helicopter because we couldn't get around any other way," explains nurse Dara. "And heaven knows, we had places to go."

We flew to the out settlement after dark, in the middle of a blinding snowstorm, a precarious flight to say the least. As we hovered a big herd of caribou comforted themselves on the landing strip. We asked them to leave. Gale force winds bounced us around, seemingly just for fun, before we landed.

I grabbed my bag of goodies and jumped onto the back of a waiting snowmobile, with a man I had never seen before, and raced to my patient.

A native man had chopped his fingers instead of the large wood pile, practically severing his fingers at the knuckles. Anything to get out of chopping wood. Everyone in the community crowded into the tentframe to see what I was going to do and I could hardly wait myself. An airtight stove provided stifling, sweltering heat against the bitter outside cold.

I provided my usual efficient emergency care, gave him Demerol for pain, and dragged him back to the chopper. The Demerol seemed to have an effect on the winds as well, for they subsided immediately. The caribou too took off for parts unknown.

A priest with flowing black robes appeared from nowhere. He asked if he could fly back with us. Before I had a chance to answer aye or nay, he plunked himself into the front passenger seat that I had my eye on. Fortunately for him, I decided to sit in the back with my patient.

As the engines roared to life a native man motioned to me from the runway. Now what. Would I take his furs to the game office for him. Without waiting for me to say aye or nay, he boarded and crammed a pile of bloody furs behind me. The stench was unbelievable.

I planned to sign up for an assertiveness training course, but my friends talked me out of it.

Lillian R. Tymchuk, RN

PLEASE TO TAKE A NUMBER
- ᴙ - ᴙ - ᴙ -

Nurse Ellen says that in the major tourist area where she works in Alberta, all kinds of things can happen.

The phone call stated that in one hour, two gastrointestinal-type patients with vomiting and diarrhea were coming in to our ER. Next phone call, make that five patients. Next phone call, make that eighteen patients.

Oriental tourists who ate some weird pasta meal got food poisoning, and came in on a bus from the Columbia Icefields. The poor wardens. They were absolutely out of their minds, because they got the worst of it when all these people got sick way up there in the campground.

I got all eighteen tourists. There's only one nurse in emergency routinely, so it was just myself, the doctor, and the ambulance attendants taking care of them. Other patients required attention as well.

I was having great difficulty with the names of the new arrivals, making it impossible to maintain any sense of order. I grabbed a stack of paper, wrote the numbers from one to eighteen down with a wide-tipped black felt pen, and taped one onto each of their chests.

My temporary system worked marvellously. After things settled down and my patients felt more comfortable, I registered each of them, taking care to spell their unfamiliar names correctly.

378

Nurse, Hear You, Hear Me

A LAW UNTO HERSELF
- ℞ - ℞ - ℞ -

"Anything that can possibly happen, happens to me. It's Murphy's Law. I'm involved in situations that most nurses never encounter." This is nurse Dotty's opinion of events that occur when she's at work in her Manitoba hospital.

The police knew me by name, what with all the teenagers going AWOL from my pediatric surgical floor. One incident concerning a male teenager stands out in my mind, although after several similar events, I began to accept them as quasi-routine.

One-to-one observation is required for attempted suicides, and for most kids involved in gang fights. One teen had fractured his hand during a fight and the police were involved. I asked one of our older aides, Helga, to sit with him. She weighed two hundred and fifty pounds and was slow to move, but she was kind and efficient.

I can always tell when the kids are getting ready to take off. They get antsy, start watching the clock, and pace around incessantly. That's exactly what this kid was doing and I instructed Helga to watch him carefully.

Around 10:00 P.M. I heard a WHOOOSH. Out of the corner of my eye I saw a thin blur in blue jeans speeding down the hall, followed by a much larger blur, huffing and puffing.

379

We laughed till we cried because we had never seen Helga move so fast — we couldn't even call a code. Like she was going to stop a six foot kid in full trot.

There is a protocol for such an event, entailing specific steps such as calling security, doing a personal check of the floor, and calling the police. Sometimes the police can track them down and bring them back.

When I called the police, the officer on duty said, "Let me guess. This is Dotty, right?"

"You got it."

Helga chased the kid deep into the bowels of the hospital, through the tunnels. Only later did she realize this was neither a smart nor safe move on her part.

The kid was gone. He virtually disappeared. He had planned his elopement well and his friends probably were waiting for him. He never did come back.

The head nurse once asked me why I didn't tell her I was a jinx. The truth of the matter is, some nurses always have quiet shifts and others always have something going on. I happen to be one of the latter. There's nothing I can do to change it. I still don't think what happened that time was such a big deal. Here's what transpired.

An eleven-year-old boy had amputated his fingers, and the plastic surgeons reattached them. The kid was put in a single room where the heat was jacked up to around ninety degrees, in an effort to enhance the circulation to the fingers.

I set the thermostat to the max and two maintenance men proudly arrived with a baseboard heater so new it was still in the box. I plugged it in and checked it out, explaining everything to my patient. The room seemed more like a sauna by the minute, and he was getting slightly uncomfortable.

A cup of tea was what I needed, and as I put the kettle on to boil, a loud and unnerving BONG-BONG-BONG rang out. The fire alarm. The fire was on our floor, according to the overhead pager.

I couldn't smell any smoke. We checked each room, including the one with the heater. Nothing.

The firemen came running in with their gas masks and tanks and checked the entire floor. They determined the problem was coming from the room with the baseboard heater, but I had already checked it to my satisfaction.

The firemen said that as the temperature of the new heater increased, it burned off the chemicals on the heater itself, causing the individual smoke alarm in the room to trigger.

"I wondered what the red light on the ceiling was," my young patient said.

The other nurse and I drew up a "Man Checklist." By the end of the night we had two cops, two maintenance men, and six firemen on the floor. But really, it wasn't such a big deal.

Lillian R. Tymchuk, RN

THE EXPERIENCED MALE
- ℞ - ℞ - ℞ -

Dina nurses in British Columbia, in a hyperbaric chamber. While modern uses of the chamber have diversified, as Dina recounts, the original intent was to treat patients with the "bends," or decompression sickness. This happens when divers go from a high pressure environment to a low pressure environment too quickly and nitrogen bubbles form in the blood.

The Cancer Control Agency has a volunteer driver program, and they pick Mrs. Jones up and drive her to our hyperbaric chamber for treatment.

Once here, she changes from street clothes into fire retardant clothing made from durette. This prevents the necessity of our asking, "What's that you're wearing? Is it polyester, is it fifty percent cotton?" Everyone wears the same thing and the resulting uniformity promotes group behaviour.

After Mrs. Jones changes she comes to the nursing station and I do a quick assessment of her vital signs, ask how she is, and how her condition has changed since her last treatment. Her co-patients are treated in a similar fashion.

There are two compartments in the hyperbaric chamber. The first one is the entry level and is ten feet long. The second one is the patient or treatment chamber, comprised of a cylindrical tube, twenty-five feet long and eight feet wide. They walk in.

Mrs. Jones takes her seat in an armchair. From one to three other patients may enter. The nurse goes in. The door is closed.

The operator starts the pressure. The pressure builds, and for the routine patients that we do every day, we simulate being thirty feet under sea water. Up to that point everything is open pressurized air. Here comes the interesting part. We deliver oxygen. Oxygen comes in and gas goes out via an exhaust valve.

Mrs. Jones secures a hood that's much like a fancy paper bag over her head and around her neck with a scarf. We inflate it with one hundred percent oxygen for her to breath. After a fifty minute period, we give her a five minute break to take the hood off and get something to drink.

The entire process is repeated. Mrs. Jones leaves the chamber, changes into her street clothes, and arranges for a ride home.

She feels exactly the same as when she came in. The oxygen she has taken in has metabolized within five minutes. Inside her body, healing of the unhealthy areas will begin.

Each condition is unique, but the average number of daily treatments is forty, from Monday to Friday. Most patients have had a spontaneous breakdown of tissue, an injury, or surgery — trauma to a specific area.

The number of divers we see today is dependent on the economy. When times are bad, we get extremely few divers with the bends, because the sport is too expensive. When times are good, we get divers who either haven't taken any courses or have forgotten what they knew.

Or it can be the experienced male who brings the inexperienced wife or girlfriend and he's going to show her what to do. She's the one who ends up running into serious trouble, and he blames her for ruining the trip.

TO HIT A WOMAN
- R - R - R -

"Various medical problems certainly can cause personality changes," says Nurse Yvonne in Ontario, "but it's also important to understand what the patient was like before the illness began."

We had a patient who had a stroke. One day I was doing his nursing care when suddenly he socked me in the chin and sent me flying across the room. As I hit the wall and slid down, an orderly who was walking by saw me and came marching in.

I thought he was going to kill this patient. I had to get up and tell him not to do anything. "You're going to get in trouble, not him," I told him, rubbing my jaw.

"Why did you hit me?" I asked my patient.

"Because I felt like it."

His history indicated a long-term abusiveness toward his current wife and two ex-wives. After his stroke, he said he hadn't hit a woman in a while, and wanted to correct the situation.

THE FINAL GIFT
- ℞ - ℞ - ℞ -

New Zealander nurse Camilla had one last experience that was destined to forever influence her nursing career in her new Alberta home.

I had been sailing for the weekend and came back to work nights. I was tanned and felt wonderful about the world after a perfect weekend out on the glorious blue waters. I had just graduated from a post-graduate intensive care course. Little did I know that I was about to look after my first organ donor.

My assignment was a twenty-three-year-old lady who had delivered her first baby. She also had a ruptured cerebral aneurysm. She was awake but clearly unstable. Her husband remained at her bedside.

She had bled, but not severely at that stage. The doctors were hoping to operate on her the following day. I was the same age as my patient, and death was not an option.

She kept saying, "We've got to name the baby," but her husband put her off. "We'll do it tomorrow when you're better," he said.

The next night she was in a coma. At report, I heard the doctors had told her husband they believed she was brain dead. I didn't really understand what brain death meant. In the morning she was to be an organ donor, but I couldn't even fathom this.

I couldn't understand how they could do this by simply asking the husband. He had spent the last two nights in the hospital because he couldn't sleep, but he went home during the daytime. Now I dreaded bumping into him. What could I possibly say? When he wasn't there I felt tremendously relieved. As I bathed this lady and got her ready for the night, my mind swirled. There must be some mistake. She couldn't be brain dead, she had a three-day-old baby. I was angry.

Her husband came in later and I couldn't understand why he would consent to organ donation, but we never spoke about it. We talked about the fact that the baby was still unnamed, and he felt he had to deal with this issue. He and his wife had selected only boys' names before.

I found this stressful. I suggested naming the baby after her mother. He said, "No, that's the name her parents gave her. My wife was given a baby and I want to name her."

He said he could never forget this month, so he called her May.

As morning drew near, I said, "I understand the doctors have spoken to you about organ donation. Do you understand what that is?"

He did. He taught me that he couldn't take his wife with him. Although she was going to die and would be buried, she could help two other people to be free of dialysis through the donation of her kidneys. He said he would have to explain to his tiny daughter who her mother was, and what better way than through her final gift. His little girl would have something to think about, something to make her proud.

Initially, I was shocked that he could even consider organ donation. After he explained it I wondered how often we didn't offer opportunities to our patients, or do certain things for them, because of our own fears and concerns. I recognized how often difficult patients have taught us what we need to know.

I realized organ donation was not my decision, but rather something we should offer to families. We could assist them if this was something they wanted to fulfill.

This experience helped me think about how I present this to families in Alberta now. I never say, "Will you consider donating your wife's organs?" I always provide it in the framework that, "Many people have considered organ and tissue donation, and if this is something you'd like to consider, I'm here to help you. If not, I'm here to help you anyway."

Today, we have a wide variety of donors. There are fewer motor vehicle accidents, but we certainly see a number of cerebral bleeds. This is a result of nature and no one is to blame.

When there is someone to blame, the remaining family members feel guilty. Suicides are difficult because families are unprepared, and the grief is made complex because of anger. We have to be careful not to feel that the anger and grief are related to organ donation. The fact is, the anger is often directed toward other areas.

Of course there are homicide cases that become donors. They are even more complex, because as well as the family, we usually have the police or the Medical Examiner involved. It's very stressful for all parties concerned.

In relation to donors, we look at the biological age and whether the organs have a normal function or not, past medical history, and other health related factors. Most kidney donors are less than seventy, although in urgent cases for liver and kidney, we're looking into the seventies.

Not too long ago our heart and lung donors used to be thirty-five years old. Now we consider them up to fifty-five or sixty. There's more knowledge available about the human body and people are healthier than they used to be.

Sometimes I'm disappointed in my own nursing colleagues when their perception of organ donation is negative, or in the way they discuss the gift of organs. That really concerns me. On the other hand, it indicates how much education we need for our colleagues.

In our practice team we emphasize the dignity of the donor. The coordinators are in the operating room and ensure the careful closure of the wound. If physicians have not closed the body neatly — this of course is a surgical procedure — we ask them to resuture. I would hate to hear from a family or funeral home that things weren't done conscientiously. I see this as part of the ongoing gift from May's mother.

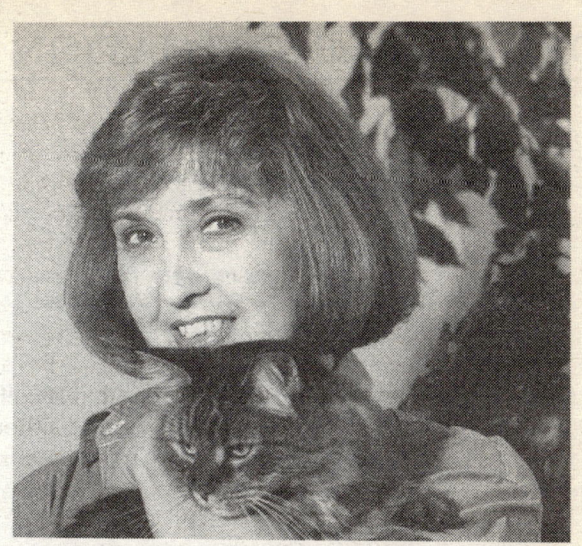

About The Author

Lillian r. Tymchuk has written numerous non-fiction articles for a variety of magazines and newspapers. She returned to McMaster University to obtain her degree in English in 1991. She was the writer for "*Homecoming '89*" which celebrated one hundred years of nursing at the Hamilton Civic Hospital.

Lillian is a registered nurse and has worked many emergency departments as head nurse, assistant supervisor, and staff nurse. She was Director of Nursing for a community based program, and also nursed in the Acquired Brain Injury Program. Prior to her nursing experience she taught with the Ontario Conservatory of Music.

ORDERING INFORMATION

Nurse Hear You, Hear Me

is great reading and would make a wonderful gift for someone you know.

To order in the United States please send cheque or money order to:

Wordstorm Productions Inc.,
1520 3rd St NW, C-104,
Great Falls, Montana, USA 59404

$8.95 + $3.50 (shipping and handling)=$12.45 (US funds)

to order in Canada please send cheque or money order to:

Wordstorm Productions Inc.,
PO Box 49132, 7740 - 18 St SE,
Calgary, Alberta, Canada T2C 3W5

$9.95 + $3.50 (shipping and handling) + $.94 (GST) + $14.39
(where applicable add HST)

PRIME CUTS: <u>65 HILARIOUS SLICES OF</u> LIFE

How does your wife get you to finish the basement? She buys you a pool table and you can't invite the guys over to play in an unfinished basement! Where do you stack freshly picked mushrooms on a hunting trip? Beside a tree of course — which looks like a million other trees in the forest. How do you calmly climb down a tree when the family cat has inserted all eighteen claws into your scalp?

This book retails for $16.95 in Canada and $14.95 in the US.

Read on and see how you can save!

<u>HOW TO ORDER</u>

In the United States: (US funds)

Tales Volume 1 - $8.95 + $3.50 (s&h) = $12.45
Tales Volume 2 - $8.95 + $3.50 (s&h) = $12.45
Prime Cuts   - $14.95 + $3.50 (s&h) = $18.45
Nurse   - $8.95 + $3.50 (s&h) = $12.45

Send Cheque or money order to:

Wordstorm Productions Inc.
1520 3rd St. NW, C-104
Great Falls, MT, USA 50404

In Canada: (CDN funds)

Tales From The Police Locker Room - Volume 1 -
$9.95+$3.50 (s&h)+$.94 (GST)= $14.39
Tales From The Police Locker Room - Volume 2 -
$9.95+ $3.50 (s&h)+$.94 (GST)= $14.39
Prime Cuts: 65 Hilarious Slices of Life - $16.95+ $3.50
(s&h)+$1.43(GST)= $21.88
Nurse - $9.95 + $3.50 (s&h) + $.94 (GST) = $14.39

(where applicable please add HST)
Mail cheque or money order to:

Wordstorm Productions Inc.,
PO Box 49132, 7740 - 18 St. SE,
Calgary, Alberta, Canada T2C 3W5

<u>Order all four books and save!</u>

In Canada:

The cost of the set is $65.05. But when you order all four books your price is only **$44.95 + $5.00** shipping and handling + 7% GST = **$53.45**, (+HST where applicable)

a savings of $11.60

In The United States:

The cost of the set is $57.80. When you order all four books your price is only **$36.95 + $5.00** shipping and handling = **$41.95**,

a savings of $15.85

(This offer expires when any or all of the titles are deemed out of print. This offer is not available in bookstores.)